INTERMITTENT FASTING DIET COOKBOOK FOR WOMEN OVER 60

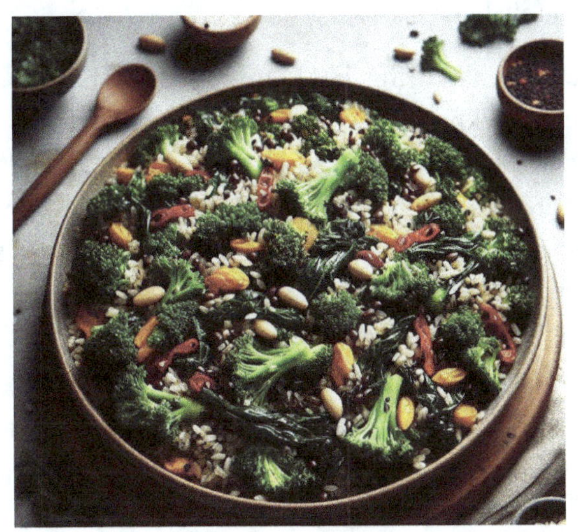

Delicious Recipes to Help You Lose Weight, Regulate Your Hormones, and Boost Metabolism

Robert Elliot

Copyright © Robert Elliot (2024)

The contents of this book are based on the author's research, knowledge, and experience. They are meant for educational purposes only and should not be taken as medical advice. Readers should consult their healthcare provider before making any changes to their health regimen.

Table of Contents

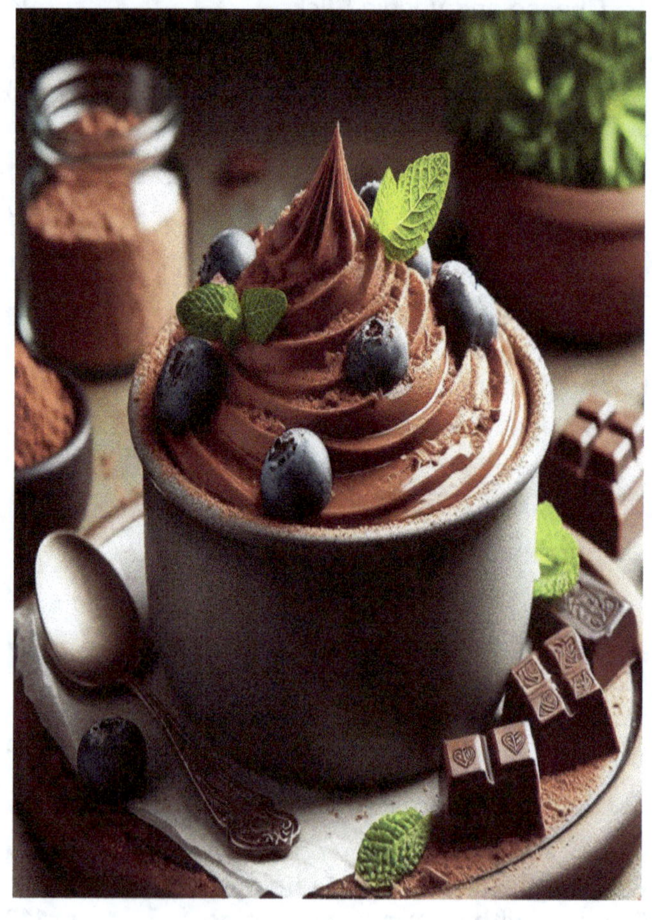

Introduction

Alright, listen up, ladies. I'm here to tell you a story. Not some fairy-tale crap, but the real deal. It's about my badass big sister, Sarah, and how she went from sugar-crazed couch potato to a walking ray of sunshine, all thanks to a little something called intermittent fasting.

Now, Sarah and I, we're cut from the same adventurous cloth. But life throws curveballs, and a few years back, Sarah wasn't hitting them out of the park. Fatigue clung to her like a bad perm. Her joints ached like rusty hinges. And don't even get me started on her sugar crashes – terrifying episodes straight out of a horror movie.

I, being the doctor and all, threw every test and pill at her. But the results were all the same: "Lifestyle adjustments needed." That's the doctor lingo for "you gotta clean up your act, sis."

Sarah, bless her stubborn heart, wasn't thrilled. But when I mentioned this "intermittent fasting" thing, something sparked in her eyes. Maybe it was the promise of no calorie counting, or the chance to ditch those afternoon sugar shakes. Whatever it was, she was in.

Now, I'm not gonna lie, the first few weeks were rough. Hunger pangs, grumpy moods, the whole shebang. But Sarah, she stuck with it. We built a support system – me whipping up her delicious low-carb meals, her cheering me on when I started running again (yes, even me!).

And then, it happened. Slowly, like a sunrise, Sarah started to change. The fatigue lifted, replaced by a spark in her eyes I hadn't seen in years. Her aches and pains faded, replaced by a newfound spring in her step. And the sugar crashes? Gone. Poof. Vanished.

But it wasn't just the physical stuff. Sarah, this woman who'd lost her zest for life, was back with a vengeance. She was taking dance classes, planning hiking trips, even writing that novel she'd always dreamt of. It was similar to watching a flower bloom after a long, hard winter.

And here's the kicker: she did it all on her own terms. No fancy shakes, no deprivation diets, just good, solid food choices and a little window of eating that fit her life.

That's why I wrote this book. Because, ladies, Sarah's story isn't hers alone. It's proof that you, too, can reclaim your health and energy, no matter your age or how stuck you feel. Intermittent fasting isn't a magic trick, but it's a powerful tool – one that unlocks the potential of your body and lets you live your best life, no matter what number hangs on the calendar.

So, are you ready to ditch the fatigue, shake off the aches, and rediscover the sparkle in your eyes? Flip the page, and let's embark on this adventure together. You won't regret it.

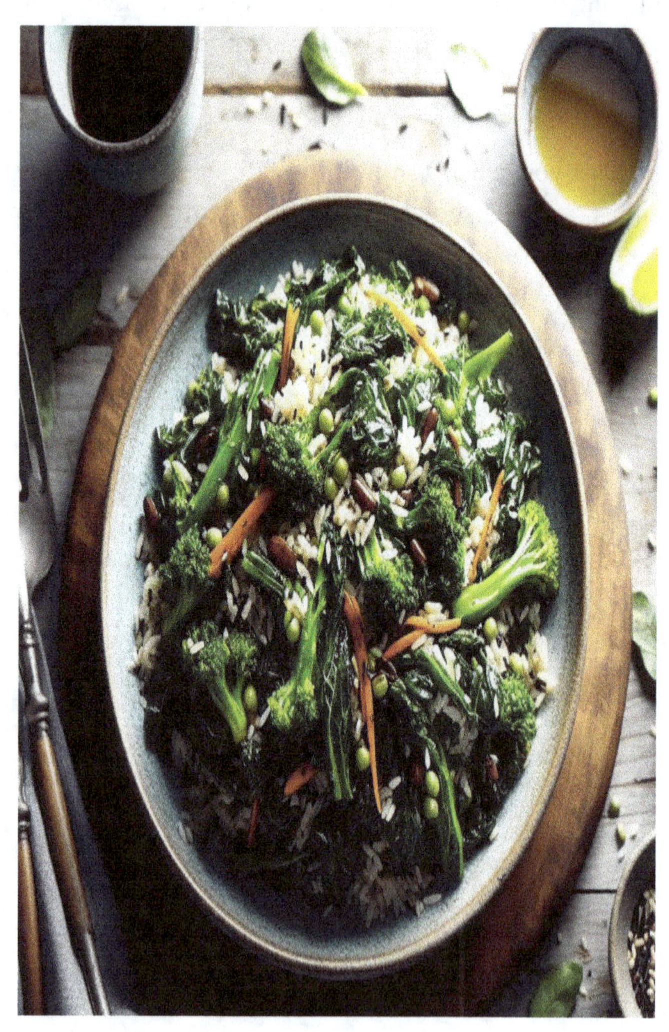

Chapter 1: Introduction to Intermittent Fasting

Welcome to a journey of discovery! This book is your guide to unlocking the potential of intermittent fasting, a dietary approach that's gaining widespread popularity for its diverse benefits, particularly for women over 60.

But before we delve into the specifics, let's take a step back and understand the core of this exciting concept.

What is Intermittent Fasting?

Intermittent fasting isn't a fad diet; it's a cyclical eating pattern that alternates between periods of eating and fasting. Unlike traditional calorie-counting diets, it focuses on **when** you eat rather than **what** you eat. This simple shift in timing can have a profound impact on your overall health and well-being.

Think of it like giving your body a break from the constant processing of food. During fasting windows, your body enters a metabolic state called ketosis, where it starts burning stored fat for energy instead of relying solely on glucose from carbohydrates. This fat-burning process can lead to a cascade of positive effects, from weight management to improved cognitive function and even reduced risk of chronic diseases.

Why is Intermittent Fasting So Appealing to Women Over 60?

As we navigate our later years, our bodies undergo natural changes. Our metabolisms slow down, hormonal fluctuations can impact weight and energy levels, and the risk of certain health conditions like diabetes and heart disease increases.

Intermittent fasting offers a powerful tool to address these challenges and empower women over 60 to thrive. Here are just a few reasons why it's resonating with this age group:

- **Weight Management**: Intermittent fasting can be a sustainable approach to weight loss or maintenance, particularly for women struggling with hormonal changes that can make weight control difficult.
- **Improved Energy Levels**: By optimizing your metabolism and burning fat for fuel, intermittent fasting can boost your energy

levels and combat fatigue, a common concern for women over 60.

- **Enhanced Cognitive Function**: Studies suggest that intermittent fasting can improve memory, focus, and cognitive function, potentially reducing the risk of age-related cognitive decline.

- **Reduced Disease Risk**: Research indicates that intermittent fasting may have protective effects against chronic diseases like type 2 diabetes, heart disease, and even certain cancers, all of which are more prevalent in older adults.

- **Cellular Repair and Longevity**: Intermittent fasting may trigger cellular repair mechanisms and promote longevity by reducing oxidative stress and inflammation in the body.

A Personalized Approach to Wellness

It's critical to keep in mind that there isn't one intermittent fasting strategy that works for everyone. There are various methods to choose from, each with its own benefits and challenges. Throughout this book, we'll explore different types of intermittent fasting and guide you in finding the approach that best aligns with your individual needs and preferences.

Safety First

Before embarking on your intermittent fasting journey, it's crucial to prioritize your health and safety. Consulting with your doctor is essential, especially if you have any underlying medical conditions or are taking medications.

This book will equip you with the knowledge and resources to make informed decisions and navigate your intermittent fasting journey with confidence. We'll delve deeper into the safety considerations and offer practical tips for ensuring a smooth and successful transition.

So, are you ready to embrace a new chapter in your health and well-being? Buckle up, grab your favorite water bottle, and let's embark on this exciting adventure together!

Chapter 2: Understanding Women's Health After 60

Our bodies are magnificent tapestries woven with the threads of time. As we reach our 60s, these threads have formed rich patterns, etched with wisdom and experience. Yet, like any living fabric, our bodies adapt and change. Understanding these changes is key to unlocking the full potential of intermittent fasting for women in this vibrant chapter of life.

Unique Nutritional Needs

1. Increased Protein Power: Maintaining muscle mass becomes crucial after 60. Protein intake becomes particularly important to combat age-related muscle loss and ensure strong bones. Aim for 0.8 grams of protein per kilogram of body weight daily. Think lean meats, fish, eggs, beans, and lentils.

2. Bone-Boosting Calcium: Bone density naturally decreases with age, increasing the risk of osteoporosis. Ensure adequate calcium intake (1,200 milligrams daily) through dairy products, leafy greens like kale and collard greens, and calcium-fortified foods.

3. Gut Health Harmony: Our gut microbiome plays a vital role in overall health, influencing digestion, immunity, and even mood. Prioritize gut-friendly foods like fermented yogurts, kefir, kimchi, and sauerkraut to nourish your good bacteria.

Addressing Common Concerns

1. Managing Menopause: Hormonal fluctuations during menopause can impact weight, energy levels, and sleep. Intermittent fasting may help regulate weight gain, improve sleep quality, and boost energy levels, offering a natural approach to managing these changes.

2. Fueling for Energy: Maintaining energy levels is crucial for an active lifestyle. Prioritize nutrient-dense whole foods, including complex carbohydrates like whole grains and fruits, healthy fats like avocado and nuts, and lean protein sources. Remember, staying hydrated is key!

3. Joint Health and Fitness: Joint pain and stiffness can become more common with age. Regular physical activity, even gentle exercises like walking or swimming, can improve joint health and flexibility. Intermittent fasting, coupled with mindful movement, can be a powerful duo for promoting physical well-being.

Intermittent Fasting: Your Ally in Health Optimization

Intermittent fasting can be a valuable tool for addressing these common concerns and promoting overall health for women over 60.

- **Weight Management**: Studies suggest that intermittent fasting can be an effective way to manage weight or lose weight, particularly for women struggling with hormonal changes.
- **Improved Insulin Sensitivity**: Intermittent fasting can improve insulin sensitivity, reducing the risk of developing type 2 diabetes, a concern for many women over 60.
- **Enhanced Cellular Repair**: The metabolic shift triggered by fasting may promote cellular repair mechanisms, potentially reducing the risk of chronic diseases and contributing to longevity.

- **Reduced Inflammation**: Chronic inflammation is linked to various health conditions. Intermittent fasting may help reduce inflammation, promoting overall well-being.

Remember, your journey is unique. Listen to your body's signals, personalize your approach to intermittent fasting, and consult with your doctor if you have any concerns.

Chapter 3: Types of Intermittent Fasting & Meal Planning

Welcome to your personal fasting playground! Now that we understand the magic behind intermittent fasting and its alignment with women's health over 60, let's explore the exciting world of its practical application. Buckle up, buttercup, because we're about to discover the perfect fasting method for your vibrant life!

A Buffet of Fasting Choices

Just like choosing ingredients for a delicious recipe, you have various "flavors" of intermittent fasting to pick from. Each offers unique benefits and challenges, so we'll dissect them one by one to help you find the perfect match for your taste buds and lifestyle.

1. Time-Restricted Eating:
Think of this method as setting boundaries for your "grazing hours." You choose a daily window for eating (e.g., 8 hours) and stick to fasting for the remaining time (e.g., 16 hours). The popular 16/8 method falls under this category, with many women finding it a natural and sustainable approach.

- **Pros**: Easy to implement, flexible, promotes fat burning, may improve sleep quality.
- **Cons**: May require adjusting meal times, initial hunger pangs are possible.

2. The 5:2 Diet:

Imagine feasting for five days and "resetting" your body with calorie restriction for two non-consecutive days. On fasting days, aim for 500-600 calories, prioritizing protein and nutrient-dense choices.

- **Pros**: Offers flexibility on eating days, potentially boosts metabolism, may improve insulin sensitivity.
- **Cons**: Requires stricter calorie counting on fasting days, may not be suitable for everyone.

3. Alternate-Day Fasting:

This method is like a flip-flop for your eating habits. You fast every other day, consuming nothing but water, black coffee, or unsweetened tea. On feasting days, enjoy healthy, balanced meals without calorie restrictions.

- **Pros**: Potentially effective for weight loss, may improve cognitive function, can be a simple to follow schedule.

- **Cons**: Can be challenging for beginners, not suitable for everyone, may induce initial hunger pangs.

4. Eat-Stop-Eat:

This method involves incorporating longer fasting periods, typically 24 hours once or twice a week. Choose non-consecutive days, listen to your body, and break your fast with a light meal like soup or salad, gradually transitioning back to regular eating.

- **Pros**: May promote cellular repair, potentially boost detoxification, offers flexibility in scheduling.
- **Cons**: Not ideal for beginners, may require initial adjustments to sleep and energy levels.

Remember: Each method has its own charm and quirks. Experiment, listen to your body, and choose the approach that suits your lifestyle and preferences. Your perfect fasting fit is out there!

Planning Your Culinary Adventure

Now that you have a diverse menu of fasting choices, let's get cooking! Meal planning is key to success, ensuring you have healthy, delicious options at your fingertips during your eating windows. Here are some tips:

- **Stock your pantry and fridge**: Focus on whole, unprocessed foods like fruits, vegetables, lean protein sources, and healthy fats.
- **Prepare grab-and-go options**: Pre-chop veggies, cook protein in advance, and have easy-to-assemble salads or bowls ready for busy mornings.
- **Embrace leftovers**: Cook larger batches and enjoy them for lunch or dinner the next day.
- **Hydration is your hero**: Keep water, unsweetened tea, and black coffee readily available during fasting windows.
- **Listen to your cravings (within reason):** If you're truly hungry during your eating window, choose satisfying yet nutritious options.

Sweetening the Journey with Delicious Recipes

Throughout this book, you'll find flavorful recipes specifically tailored for intermittent fasting, catering to various dietary preferences and taste buds. From satisfying salads and protein-packed bowls to comforting soups and light yet fulfilling stir-fries, we'll fuel your journey with delectable delights.

In the next chapter, we'll explore delicious intermittent fasting-tailored breakfast recipes that will leave your taste bud buzzing.

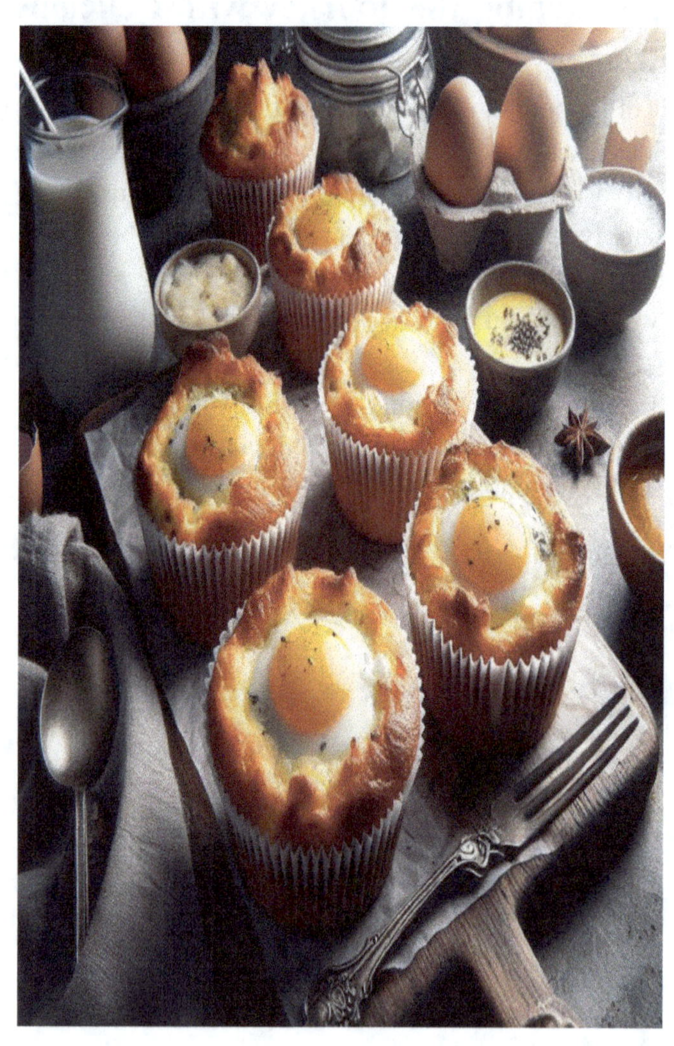

Chapter 4: Breakfast

Almond Flour Pancakes

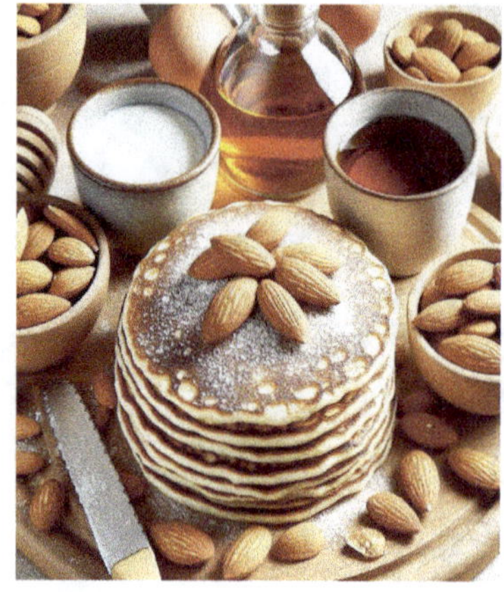

Preparation Time: 10 minutes
Cooking Time: 10-12 minutes
Servings: 6-8 pancakes

Ingredients:
- 1 cup almond flour
- 2 tbsp coconut flour
- 1/2 tsp baking powder
- 1/4 tsp baking soda
- 1/4 tsp salt
- 1 egg
- 1 cup unsweetened almond milk
- 1 tsp vanilla extract
- 1 tbsp melted coconut oil

Directions:
1. In a large bowl, whisk together the almond flour, coconut flour, baking powder, baking soda, and salt.

2. In a separate bowl, whisk together the egg, almond milk, vanilla extract, and melted coconut oil.

3. Pour the wet ingredients into the dry ingredients and whisk until just combined. Don't overmix!

4. Heat a lightly greased griddle or frying pan over medium heat.

5. Pour batter onto the griddle, forming 2-3 inch pancakes.

6. Cook for 2-3 minutes per side, or until golden brown and cooked through.

7. Serve warm with your favorite toppings, such as maple syrup, fresh fruit, or nuts.

Nutritional Values per Serving:
Calories: 180 | Carbs: 8g | Fat: 13g
Fiber: 4g | Protein: 9g | Sugar: 3g

Hearty Pancakes

Preparation Time: 10 minutes
Cooking Time: 15-20 minutes
Servings: 4-6 pancakes

Ingredients:
- 1 cup whole wheat flour
- 1/2 cup rolled oats
- 1 tsp baking powder
- 1/2 tsp baking soda
- 1/4 tsp salt
- 1 cup milk
- 1 egg
- 1 tbsp honey
- 1 tbsp olive oil

Directions:
1. In a large bowl, whisk together the flour, oats, baking powder, baking soda, and salt.
2. In a separate bowl, whisk together the milk, egg, honey, and olive oil.
3. After adding the wet ingredients to the dry ones, mix until just combined. Fold in any desired mix-ins, such as chopped nuts, berries, or shredded vegetables.

4. Heat a lightly greased griddle or frying pan over medium heat.

5. Pour batter onto the griddle, forming 4-inch pancakes.

6. Cook for 3-4 minutes per side, or until golden brown and cooked through.

7. Serve warm with your favorite toppings, such as yogurt, nuts, or a drizzle of maple syrup.

Nutritional Values per Serving:
Calories: 250 | Carbs: 29g | Fat: 10g
Fiber: 5g | Protein: 12g | Sugar: 7g

Egg Muffins

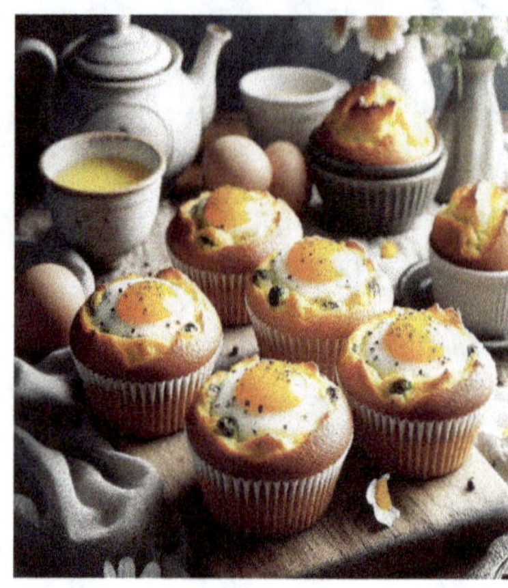

Preparation Time: 10 minutes
Cooking Time: 20-25 minutes
Servings: 12 muffins

Ingredients:
- 12 eggs
- 1/2 cup chopped vegetables (e.g., bell peppers, spinach, mushrooms)
- 1/4 cup crumbled cooked sausage or bacon (optional)
- 1/4 cup shredded cheese
- Salt and pepper to taste

Directions:
1. Preheat oven to 350°F (175°C).
2. Grease a muffin tin with 12 wells.

3. Divide the vegetables, sausage or bacon (if using), and cheese evenly among the muffin cups.

4. Whisk together the eggs and season with salt and pepper.

5. Pour the egg mixture into the muffin cups, filling each one almost to the top.

6. Bake for 20-25 minutes, or until the eggs are set and cooked through.

7. Let cool slightly before serving.

Nutritional Values per Serving (1 Muffin):
Calories: 100 | Carbs: 1g | Fat: 7g |
Fiber: 1g | Protein: 7g | Sugar: 1g

Pomegranate Quinoa Porridge

Preparation Time: 5 minutes
Cooking Time: 15 minutes
Servings: 2

Ingredients:
- 1/2 cup cooked quinoa
- 1 cup unsweetened almond milk
- 1/4 cup pomegranate juice
- 1/4 teaspoon ground cinnamon
- 1/4 cup pomegranate arils
- 1 tablespoon chopped almonds (optional)
- Maple syrup or honey to taste (optional)

Directions:

1. In a saucepan, combine cooked quinoa, almond milk, pomegranate juice, and cinnamon.

2. Bring to a simmer over medium heat and cook for 10-15 minutes, stirring occasionally, until thickened and creamy.

3. Remove from heat and stir in pomegranate arils and almonds (if using).

4. Serve warm with honey or maple syrup, if desired.

Tips:
- For a richer flavor, use coconut milk instead of almond milk.
- You can also add other toppings like chopped nuts, berries, or a drizzle of tahini.
- You may keep leftovers in the fridge for up to three days.

Pineapple Oatmeal

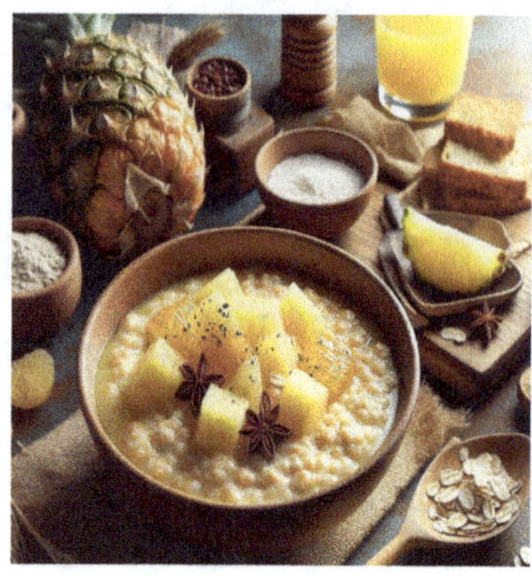

Preparation Time: 5 minutes
Cooking Time: 10 minutes
Servings: 2

Ingredients:
- 1/2 cup rolled oats
- 1 cup water or milk
- 1/4 cup chopped fresh pineapple
- 1/4 teaspoon ground cinnamon
- 1/4 teaspoon ground ginger
- 1 tablespoon chopped walnuts (optional)
- Maple syrup or honey to taste (optional)

Directions:

1. In a saucepan, combine oats, water or milk, pineapple, cinnamon, and ginger.

2. Bring to a boil over medium heat, then reduce heat and simmer for 10 minutes, stirring occasionally, until thickened.

3. Remove from heat and stir in walnuts (if using).

4. Serve warm with honey or maple syrup, if desired.

Nutritional Values per Serving:
Calories: 200 | Carbs: 31g | Fat: 4g |
Fiber: 4g | Protein: 5g | Sugar: 10g

Tips:

- If fresh pineapple isn't available, use canned pineapple chunks.

- You can also add other toppings like chopped berries, coconut flakes, or seeds.

- You may keep leftovers in the fridge for up to three days.

Waffles with Whipped Cream

Preparation Time: 10 minutes (plus waffle batter preparation time)
Cooking Time: 5-7 minutes per waffle
Servings: 2-3 (depending on waffle size)

Ingredients:
- **2-3 cups prepared waffle batter (made according to your preferred recipe)**
- **1 cup whipped cream**
- **Fresh fruit (optional)**
- **Maple syrup or other toppings (optional)**

Directions:
1. As directed by the manufacturer, preheat your waffle iron.
2. Pour batter into the waffle iron and cook until golden brown and crispy, about 5-7 minutes.
3. While the waffles are cooking, prepare your whipped cream. You can use store-bought whipped cream or make your own by whipping heavy cream with a hand mixer or whisk until stiff peaks form.
4. Serve waffles warm with whipped cream and your favorite toppings.

Tips:
- For a healthier option, use whole-grain waffle batter.
- You can top your waffles with fresh fruit, nuts, seeds, or a drizzle of maple syrup or honey.
- Leftover waffles can be stored in the freezer for up to 3 months and reheated in the toaster or oven.

Tomato and Egg Scramble

Preparation Time: 5 minutes
Cooking Time: 10 minutes
Servings: 2

Ingredients:
- 2 eggs
- 1/2 medium tomato, diced
- 1/4 cup chopped onion
- 1 tablespoon olive oil
- Salt and pepper to taste
- Fresh herbs (optional, such as parsley, basil, or chives)

Directions:
1. In a bowl, whisk together the eggs.
2. In a frying pan, warm the olive oil over medium heat. After adding, simmer for three minutes, or until the onion is tender.
3. Add the diced tomato and cook for another 2-3 minutes, until slightly softened.
4. Pour in the whisked eggs and scramble until cooked through, about 5 minutes.
5. Add salt and pepper to your desired taste.
6. Garnish with fresh herbs, if desired.

Tips:

- Add a tablespoon of grated Parmesan cheese for a richer flavor.

- You can also add other vegetables to the scramble, such as spinach, mushrooms, or bell peppers.

- Leftover scramble can be stored in the refrigerator for up to 2 days.

Mexican Avocado Salad

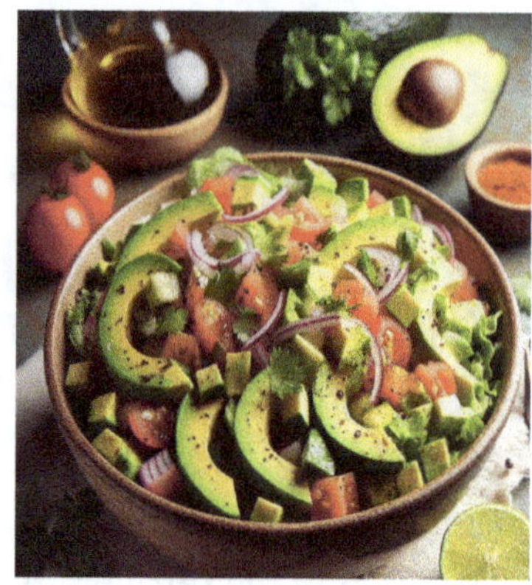

Preparation Time: 10 minutes
Cooking Time: None
Servings: 1-2

Ingredients:
- 1 ripe avocado, halved and pitted
- 1/2 cup diced tomatoes
- 1/4 cup chopped red onion
- 1/4 cup chopped cilantro
- 1/4 cup crumbled feta cheese
- 1 tablespoon lime juice
- 1/2 teaspoon chili powder
- Salt and pepper to taste

Directions:

1. Scoop out the avocado flesh and mash it in a bowl.

2. Add the diced tomatoes, red onion, cilantro, feta cheese, lime juice, chili powder, salt, and pepper.

3. Stir to combine.

4. Serve immediately, topped with a fried egg (optional).

Nutritional Values per Serving:
Calories: 300 | Carbs: 10g | Fat: 20g |
Fiber: 5g | Protein: 8g | Sugar: 2g

Tips:

- This salad can be made ahead of time and stored in the refrigerator for up to 1 day.

- Add a pinch of cayenne pepper for a spicier flavor.

- You can also serve this salad on a bed of lettuce or with tortilla chips.

Chili Omelet

Preparation Time: 10 minutes
Cooking Time: 15 minutes
Servings: 1-2

Ingredients:
- 2 eggs
- 1/4 cup cooked and crumbled ground beef or chili
- 1/4 cup shredded cheddar cheese
- 1/4 cup chopped tomato
- 1/4 cup chopped onion
- 1 tablespoon olive oil
- Salt and pepper to taste

Directions:
1. In a bowl, whisk together the eggs.
2. In a frying pan, warm the olive oil over medium heat. After adding, simmer for 3 minutes, or until the onion is tender.
3. Add the cooked ground beef or chili and cook for another 2 minutes.
4. Pour in the whisked eggs and scramble until almost cooked through.
5. Sprinkle with cheddar cheese and tomato.

6. Fold the omelet in half and cook for another minute or two, until the cheese is melted.

7. Add salt and pepper to suit your taste.

Nutritional Values per Serving:
Calories: 350 | Carbs: 4g | Fat: 25g |
Fiber: 1g | Protein: 20g | Sugar: 2g

Tips:

- You can use leftover chili or taco meat in this recipe.

- For a lighter option, use ground turkey or chicken.

- You can also add other vegetables to the omelet, such as spinach, mushrooms, or bell peppers.

Flavorful Pumpkin Pie Oatmeal

Preparation Time: 5 minutes
Cooking Time: 15 minutes
Servings: 2

Ingredients:
- 1/2 cup rolled oats
- 1 cup water or unsweetened almond milk
- 1/4 cup cooked pumpkin puree
- 1/4 teaspoon pumpkin pie spice
- 1/4 teaspoon ground cinnamon
- 1 tablespoon chopped walnuts or pecans (optional)
- Maple syrup or honey to taste (optional)

Directions:
1. In a saucepan, combine the oats, almond milk or water, pumpkin puree, pumpkin pie spice, and cinnamon.
2. Bring to a boil over medium heat, then reduce heat and simmer for 10-15 minutes, stirring occasionally, until thickened and creamy.
3. Remove from heat and stir in the nuts (if using).
4. Serve warm with maple syrup or honey, if desired.

Nutritional Values per Serving:
Calories: 250 | Carbs: 30g | Fat: 5g |
Fiber: 5g | Protein: 5g | Sugar: 7g

Tips:

- For a richer flavor, use full-fat coconut milk instead of almond milk.

- You can add other toppings like chopped fruit, dried cranberries, or a dollop of yogurt.

- You can keep leftovers in the fridge for three days or longer.

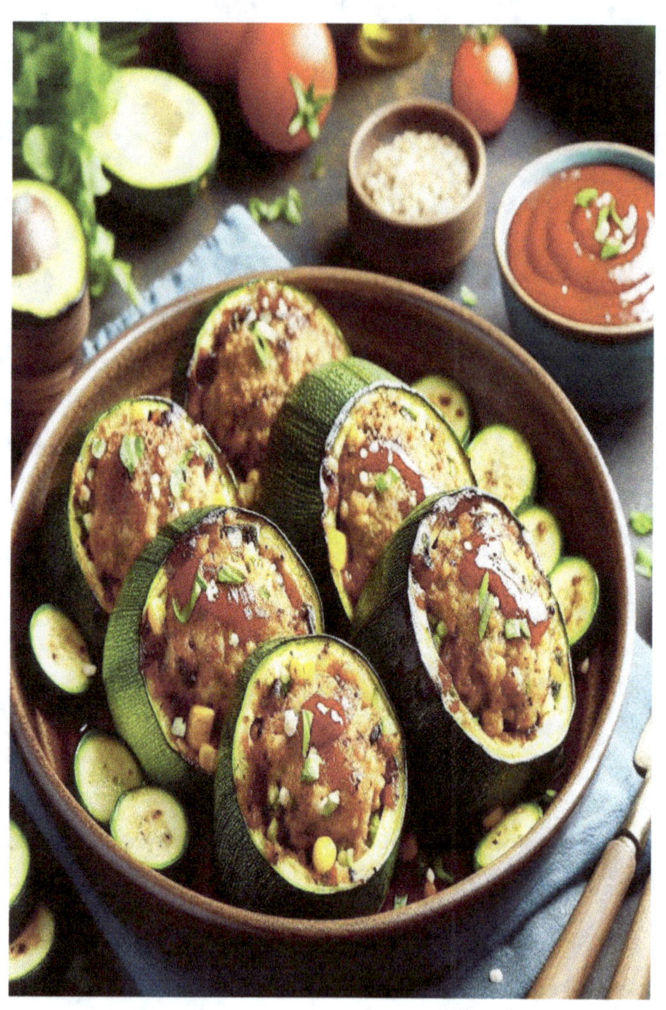

Chapter 5: Lunch

Kale and Wild Rice Stir Fry

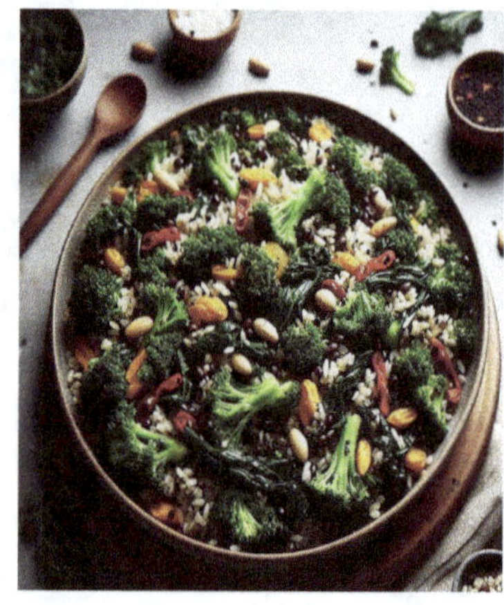

Preparation Time: 15 minutes
Cooking Time: 20 minutes
Servings: 4

Ingredients:
- 1 tablespoon olive oil
- 1/2 cup chopped onion
- 2 cloves garlic, minced
- 5 cups chopped kale
- 1 cup cooked wild rice
- 1/2 cup vegetable broth
- 1/4 cup low-sodium soy sauce
- 1 tablespoon maple syrup
- 1 teaspoon sriracha (optional)
- Sesame seeds and sliced almonds, for garnish

Directions:

1. Heat olive oil in a large wok or frying pan over medium heat. Simmer the onion and garlic for 3 minutes, or until they are tender.

2. Add kale and cook until wilted, about 5 minutes.

3. Stir in cooked wild rice, vegetable broth, soy sauce, maple syrup, and sriracha (if using).

4. Cook for another 5 minutes, until heated through.

5. Serve garnished with sesame seeds and sliced almonds.

Nutritional Values per Serving:
Calories: 350 | Carbs: 39g | Fat: 10g |
Fiber: 6g | Protein: 15g | Sugar: 8g

Tips:

- You can use any type of cooked rice in this recipe, such as brown rice or quinoa.

- Feel free to add other vegetables to the stir fry, such as carrots, bell peppers, or mushrooms.

- For a heartier meal, serve the stir fry over a bed of cooked brown rice or quinoa.

Zucchini Omelet

Preparation Time: 10 minutes
Cooking Time: 15 minutes
Servings: 1-2

Ingredients:
- 2 eggs
- 1/2 medium zucchini, grated
- 1/4 cup chopped onion
- 1 tablespoon olive oil
- Salt and pepper to taste
- Fresh herbs (optional, such as parsley, basil, or chives)

Directions:
1. In a bowl, whisk together the eggs.
2. Squeeze off any extra moisture after grating the zucchini.
3. In a frying pan over medium heat, warm the olive oil. After adding, simmer for 3 minutes, or until the onion is tender.
4. Add the grated zucchini and cook for another 5 minutes, until softened.
5. Pour in the whisked eggs and scramble until cooked through, about 5 minutes.

6. Add salt and pepper to your desired taste.
7. Garnish with fresh herbs, if desired.

Nutritional Values per Serving:
Calories: 200 | Carbs: 3g | Fat: 12g |
Fiber: 2g | Protein: 14g | Sugar: 2g

Tips:
- For a lighter option, use egg whites instead of whole eggs.
- Leftover omelet can be stored in the refrigerator for up to 2 days and reheated in the microwave or on the stovetop.

Steamed Vegetable Pan

Preparation Time: 10 minutes
Cooking Time: 15 minutes
Servings: 4

Ingredients:
- 1 tablespoon olive oil
- 1/2 cup chopped onion
- 2 cloves garlic, minced
- 1 cup broccoli florets
- 1 cup chopped carrots
- 1 cup green beans, trimmed and snapped
- 1/2 cup chopped bell pepper
- 1/4 cup water
- 1/4 teaspoon dried thyme
- Salt and pepper to taste

Directions:
1. In a big skillet or wok over medium heat, warm up the olive oil. Simmer the onion and garlic for 3 minutes, or until they are tender.
2. Add broccoli, carrots, green beans, and bell pepper.
3. Pour in water and sprinkle with thyme.

4. Cover and steam for 10-15 minutes, or until vegetables are tender-crisp.

5. Season with salt and pepper to taste.

Nutritional Values per Serving:
Calories: 150 | Carbs: 10g | Fat: 5g |
Fiber: 5g | Protein: 3g | Sugar: 5g

Tips:

- Feel free to add other vegetables to this recipe, such as asparagus, zucchini, or mushrooms.

- You can also add a protein source, such as grilled chicken or shrimp, to make this a more complete meal.

- Serve this steamed vegetable pan with a side of brown rice or quinoa for a satisfying lunch.

Low Carb Stuffed Zucchini and BBQ

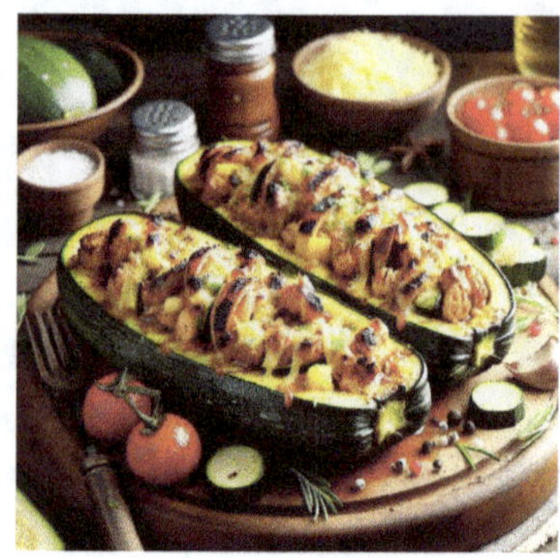

Preparation Time: 20 minutes
Cooking Time: 20 minutes
Servings: 4

Ingredients:
- 2 medium zucchini, halved lengthwise
- 1 tablespoon olive oil
- 1/2 cup chopped onion
- 2 cloves garlic, minced
- 1/2 cup ground beef or turkey
- 1/4 cup chopped tomatoes
- 1/4 cup diced bell pepper
- 1/4 cup shredded cheddar cheese
- 1/4 cup low-carb BBQ sauce

Directions:

1. Preheat oven to 400°F (200°C).

2. Scoop out the flesh from the zucchini halves, leaving a 1/2-inch border. Dice the zucchini flesh and set aside.

3. Heat olive oil in a skillet over medium heat. Simmer the onion and garlic for three minutes, or until they are tender.
4. Add ground beef or turkey and cook until browned.
5. Stir in diced zucchini flesh, tomatoes, and bell pepper. Cook for another 5 minutes.
6. Remove from heat and stir in cheddar cheese and 2 tablespoons of the BBQ sauce.
7. Spoon the mixture into the zucchini halves.
8. Top with remaining BBQ sauce.
9. Bake for 20 minutes, or until zucchini is tender and cheese is melted.

Nutritional Values per Serving:
Calories: 300 | Carbs: 7g | Fat: 20g |
Fiber: 3g | Protein: 25g | Sugar: 5g

Tips:
- You can use ground chicken or sausage instead of ground beef or turkey.
- Feel free to add other vegetables to the stuffing, such as mushrooms, spinach, or zucchini.
- Serve these stuffed zucchini halves with a side of low-carb salad or green beans.

Salmon and Green Beans

Preparation Time: 10 minutes
Cooking Time: 15 minutes
Servings: 2

Ingredients:
- 2 salmon fillets (6 oz each)
- 1 tablespoon olive oil
- 1/2 teaspoon dried thyme
- Salt and pepper to taste
- 1 pound fresh green beans, trimmed
- 1/4 cup lemon juice
- 1 tablespoon chopped fresh parsley (optional)

Directions:
1. Preheat oven to 400°F (200°C).
2. Using paper towels, pat the salmon fillets dry. Add a drizzle of olive oil and season with pepper, salt, and thyme.
3. Transfer the salmon to a baking sheet and bake it for ten to fifteen minutes, or until it is cooked through.
4. While the salmon is cooking, bring a pot of salted water to a boil. Add the green beans and cook for 3-5 minutes, or until tender-crisp.

5. Drain the green beans and toss with lemon juice and parsley (if using).

6. Serve the salmon with the green beans, enjoying the perfectly cooked fish and vibrant vegetables.

Nutritional Values per Serving:
Calories: 400 | Carbs: 11g | Fat: 25g |
Fiber: 4g | Protein: 35g | Sugar: 2g

Tips:

- You can also cook the salmon on the grill or in a stovetop pan.

- Feel free to add other vegetables to the side dish, such as broccoli, asparagus, or zucchini.

- For a richer flavor, serve the salmon with a dollop of pesto or a squeeze of lemon juice.

Toasted and Grilled Pecan Vinaigrette

Preparation Time: 10 minutes
Cooking Time: 7 minutes
Servings: 4

Ingredients:
- 1/4 cup extra virgin olive oil
- 2 tablespoons red wine vinegar
- 1 tablespoon Dijon mustard
- 1/2 teaspoon honey
- 1/4 teaspoon dried thyme
- Salt and pepper to taste
- 1/4 cup chopped pecans
- 2 tablespoons chopped red onion

Directions:

1. In a small bowl, whisk together olive oil, red wine vinegar, Dijon mustard, honey, thyme, salt, and pepper.

2. Heat a dry skillet over medium heat. Add the pecans and toast for 5 minutes, stirring occasionally, until golden brown.

3. Add the red onion to the skillet and cook for another 2 minutes, until softened.

4. Transfer the pecan mixture to the bowl with the vinaigrette and stir to combine.

5. This versatile vinaigrette can be used on salads, grilled chicken or fish, or as a dipping sauce for crudités.

Nutritional Values per Serving:
Calories: 150 | Carbs: 4g | Fat: 12g |
Fiber: 1g | Protein: 1g | Sugar: 3g

Tips:

- You can use any type of nuts in this recipe, such as walnuts, almonds, or pistachios.

- Feel free to add other herbs to the vinaigrette, such as parsley, basil, or chives.

- This vinaigrette can be stored in the refrigerator for up to 1 week.

Lean Beef Vegetable Soup

Preparation Time: 15 minutes
Cooking Time: 1 hour
Servings: 6

Ingredients:
- 1 pound lean ground beef
- 1 tablespoon olive oil
- 1 medium onion, chopped
- 2 cloves garlic, minced
- 4 cups low-sodium beef broth
- 1 (14.5 oz) can diced tomatoes, undrained
- 1 (15 oz) can kidney beans, drained and rinsed
- 1 (15 oz) can corn, drained
- 1 cup chopped carrots
- 1 cup chopped celery
- 1/2 cup chopped green beans
- 1/2 teaspoon dried thyme
- Salt and pepper to taste

Directions:
1. In a large Dutch oven or pot, brown the ground beef over medium heat, draining off any excess fat.
2. Add the olive oil, onion, and garlic and cook until softened, about 5 minutes.

3. Stir in the beef broth, diced tomatoes, kidney beans, corn, carrots, celery, green beans, and thyme.
4. Bring to a boil, then reduce heat to low and simmer for 45 minutes, or until vegetables are tender.
5. Season with salt and pepper to suit your taste.

Nutritional Values per Serving (approximate):
Calories: 300 | Carbs: 30g | Fat: 15g |
Fiber: 5g | Protein: 25g | Sugar: 1g

Tips:
- This hearty and flavorful soup is packed with protein and vegetables, making it a perfect lunch option.
- Serve it with a side of whole-wheat bread or crackers for a complete meal.

Chicken Breast with Pan Vegetables

Preparation Time: 15 minutes
Cooking Time: 20 minutes
Servings: 4

Ingredients:
- 4 boneless, skinless chicken breasts
- 1 tablespoon olive oil
- Salt and pepper to taste
- 1/2 cup chopped onion
- 2 cloves garlic, minced
- 1 bell pepper, sliced
- 1 cup broccoli florets
- 1/2 cup cherry tomatoes
- 1/4 cup chicken broth
- 1/4 cup chopped fresh parsley (optional)

Directions:
1. Preheat oven to 400°F (200°C).
2. Sprinkle salt and pepper on the chicken breasts.
3. Heat olive oil in a large ovenproof skillet over medium heat. Sear the chicken breasts on both sides until golden brown, about 5 minutes per side.

4. Transfer the skillet to the oven and bake for 10-15 minutes, or until the chicken is cooked through.

5. While the chicken is cooking, add the onion, garlic, bell pepper, and broccoli to the skillet and cook for 5 minutes, or until softened.

6. Stir in the cherry tomatoes and chicken broth. Bring to a simmer and cook for another 5 minutes, or until the vegetables are tender and the tomatoes have burst.

7. Garnish with chopped parsley (if using) and serve the chicken with the pan vegetables.

Nutritional Values per Serving:
**Calories: 350 | Carbs: 11g | Fat: 20g |
Fiber: 4g | Protein: 35g | Sugar: 5g**

Tips:

- You can use any type of vegetables in this recipe, such as zucchini, asparagus, or mushrooms.

- Feel free to add a bit of spice to the dish with a pinch of chili flakes or cayenne pepper.

- Serve this dish with a side of brown rice or quinoa for a more complete meal.

Sweet Corn Soup

Preparation Time: 10 minutes
Cooking Time: 20 minutes
Servings: 4

Ingredients:
- 1 tablespoon olive oil
- 1/2 cup chopped onion
- 2 cloves garlic, minced
- 4 cups frozen corn kernels
- 4 cups low-sodium chicken broth
- 1/2 cup heavy cream (optional)
- Salt and pepper to taste
- Fresh herbs (optional, such as basil, parsley, or chives)

Directions:

1. In a big saucepan, warm up the olive oil over medium heat. Add onion and garlic and cook until softened, about 5 minutes.

2. Add the frozen corn kernels and chicken broth. Bring to a boil, then reduce heat to low and simmer for 15 minutes.

3. Remove from heat and let cool slightly. Use an immersion blender or a blender in batches to puree the soup until it's smooth.

4. Stir in the heavy cream (if using) and season with salt and pepper to taste.

5. Garnish with fresh herbs (if using) and serve hot.

Nutritional Values per Serving:
Calories: 250 | Carbs: 25g | Fat: 10g |
Fiber: 5g | Protein: 5g | Sugar: 10g

Tips:

- For this dish, fresh or frozen corn kernels can be used.

- For a thicker soup, use less chicken broth or puree part of the soup and stir it back in.

- Feel free to add other vegetables to the soup, such as carrots, potatoes, or zucchini.

- This soup can be served hot or cold.

Yogurt Sauce with Chicken Souvlaki

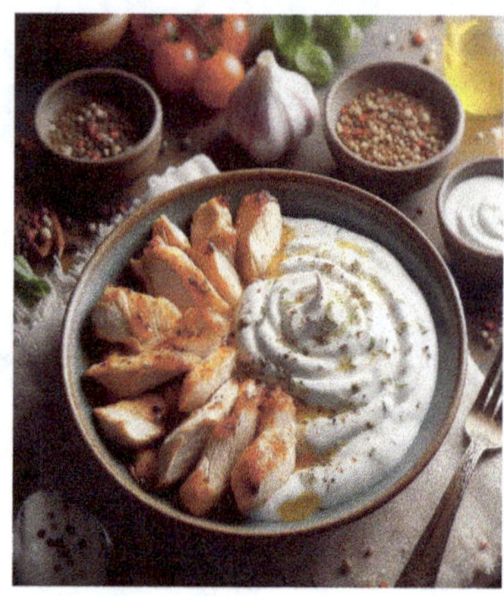

Preparation Time: 10 minutes
Cooking Time: 15 minutes (chicken)
Servings: 4

Ingredients:
Yogurt Sauce:
- 1 cup plain Greek yogurt (2% fat)
- 2 tablespoons olive oil
- 1/2 lemon, juiced
- 1 clove garlic, minced
- 1/4 teaspoon dried oregano
- Salt and pepper to taste

Chicken Souvlaki:
- 1 pound skinless, boneless chicken thighs or breasts, diced into 1-inch cubes
- 1/4 cup olive oil
- 2 tablespoons lemon juice

- 1 tablespoon red wine vinegar
- 1 tablespoon dried oregano
- 1 teaspoon garlic powder
- 1/2 teaspoon salt
- 1/4 teaspoon black pepper
- 8 wooden skewers

Directions:

1. Combine yogurt, olive oil, lemon juice, garlic, oregano, salt, and pepper in a bowl.

2. Whisk until smooth and set aside.

3. In another bowl, combine olive oil, lemon juice, red wine vinegar, oregano, garlic powder, salt, and pepper.

4. Include the cubed chicken and toss to coat. Marinate for a minimum of 30 minutes and a maximum of 4 hours.

5. Prepare your grill or broiler for medium-high heat. If using skewers, soak them in water for 30 minutes to prevent burning.

6. Thread chicken cubes onto skewers. Bake or grill for 5 to 7 minutes on each side, or until well done.

7. Enjoy the flavorful chicken with the refreshing yogurt sauce. You can also serve it with pita bread, chopped tomatoes, onions, cucumber, and crumbled feta cheese.

Chicken Souvlaki:
Calories: 300 | Carbs: 4g | Fat: 15g |
Fiber: 1g | Protein: 30g | Sugar: 1g

Chapter 6: Dinner

Chicken Skewers with Rosemary Buttermilk

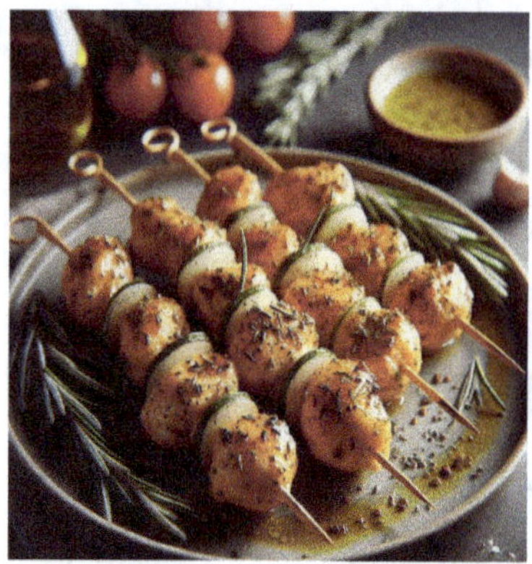

Preparation Time: 10 minutes
Marinating Time: 2 hours or overnight
Cooking Time: 15 minutes
Servings: 4

Ingredients:

- 1 pound skinless, boneless chicken thighs or breasts, diced into 1-inch cubes
- 1 cup buttermilk
- 2 tablespoons chopped fresh rosemary
- 1 teaspoon garlic powder
- 1/2 teaspoon salt
- 1/4 teaspoon black pepper
- 8 wooden skewers

Directions:

1. In a bowl, combine buttermilk, rosemary, garlic powder, salt, and pepper. Add the chicken cubes and toss to coat.

2. For optimal taste, marinate for at least two hours or overnight.

3. Prepare your grill or broiler for medium-high heat. If using skewers, soak them in water for 30 minutes to prevent burning.

4. Thread chicken cubes onto skewers. Bake or grill for 5 to 7 minutes on each side, or until well done.

5. Pair the rosemary-infused chicken with your favorite dipping sauce, grilled vegetables, or a side salad for a balanced meal.

Nutritional Values per Serving (approx.):
Calories: 250 | Carbs: 2g | Fat: 10g |
Fiber: 1g | Protein: 30g | Sugar: 1g

Zucchini Pasta With Pesto Sauce

Prep Time: 10 minutes | Cooking Time: 5 minutes | Servings: 2

Ingredients:
- 2 medium zucchini, spiralized or julienned
- 1/2 cup pesto sauce (choose your favorite variety)
- 1/4 cup cherry tomatoes, halved
- 1/4 cup crumbled feta cheese
- Fresh basil leaves, for garnish
- Salt and pepper to taste

Directions:
1. Steam or sauté the zucchini noodles until tender-crisp, about 3-5 minutes.
2. Toss the cooked zucchini noodles with pesto sauce, cherry tomatoes, feta cheese, and fresh basil.
3. Season with salt and pepper to taste.
4. Enjoy a light and flavorful vegetarian or gluten-free pasta alternative.

Nutritional Values per Serving (approx.):
Calories: 200 | Carbs: 12g | Fat: 10g | Fiber: 3g | Protein: 5g | Sugar: 5g

---

Veggie Black Bean Burger

Preparation Time: 15 minutes
Cooking Time: 20 minutes (including grilling)
Servings: 4

Ingredients:
- 1 (15 oz) can, rinsed and drained black beans
- 1 cup grated carrots
- 1/2 cup chopped bell pepper (any color)
- 1/4 cup chopped onion
- 1/4 cup rolled oats
- 1/4 cup chopped fresh cilantro
- 1 tablespoon olive oil
- 1 teaspoon ground cumin
- 1/2 teaspoon chili powder
- 1/4 teaspoon garlic powder
- Salt and pepper to taste
- Hamburger buns and desired toppings (lettuce, tomato, onion, avocado, etc.)

Directions:
1. Prepare your grill or skillet for medium heat.
2. In a bowl, mash the black beans with a fork, leaving some chunks. Add the grated carrots, bell pepper, onion, oats, cilantro, olive oil, cumin, chili

powder, garlic powder, salt, and pepper. Mix well to combine.

3. Divide the mixture into 4 equal portions and shape into patties.

4. Grill or pan-fry the patties for 5-7 minutes per side, or until cooked through and slightly firm.

5. Assemble your burgers on buns with your favorite toppings. Enjoy a hearty and healthy meatless option.

Nutritional Values per Serving (approx.):
Calories: 250 | Carbs: 24g | Fat: 7g |
Fiber: 6g | Protein: 15g | Sugar: 5g

Avocado Salsa with Grilled Salmon

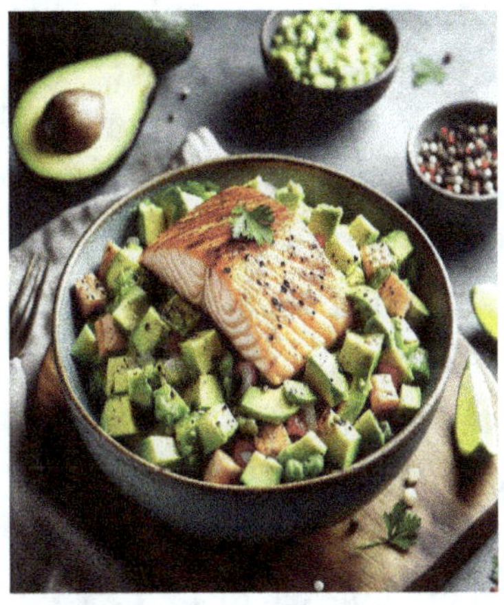

Preparation Time: 15 minutes
Cooking Time: 10 minutes (salmon)
Servings: 2

Ingredients:

Salsa:

- 1 ripe avocado, diced
- 1/2 cup chopped red onion
- 1/4 cup chopped fresh cilantro
- 1 lime, juiced
- 1/4 teaspoon chili powder
- Salt and pepper to taste

Salmon:

- 2 salmon fillets (6 oz each)
- 1 tablespoon olive oil
- 1/2 teaspoon dried dill
- 1/4 teaspoon garlic powder

- Salt and pepper to taste

Directions:
1. Combine diced avocado, red onion, cilantro, lime juice, chili powder, salt, and pepper in a bowl. Set aside.
2. In a separate bowl, toss the salmon fillets with olive oil, dill, garlic powder, salt, and pepper.
3. Prepare your grill or broiler for medium-high heat.
4. Grill or broil the salmon fillets for 5-7 minutes per side, or until cooked through and lightly flaked.
5. Top the cooked salmon with the avocado salsa and enjoy a flavorful and protein-rich dish.

Nutritional Values per Serving (approx.):
Calories: 400 | Carbs: 7g | Fat: 25g |
Fiber: 3g | Protein: 35g | Sugar: 3g

Keto Wraps with Cream Cheese and Salmon

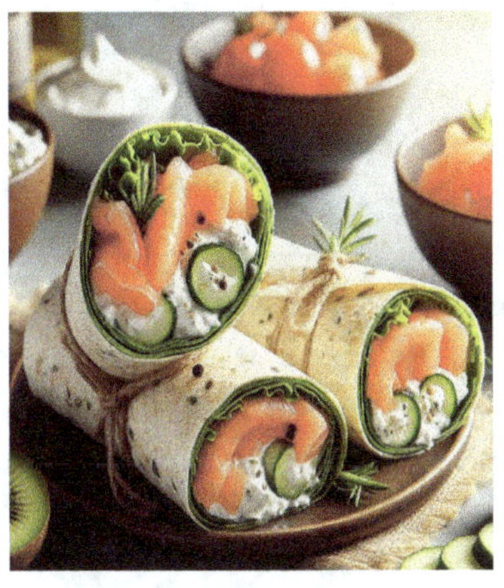

Preparation Time: 10 minutes
Cooking Time: 5 minutes (optional)
Servings: 2

Ingredients:
- 2 large romaine lettuce leaves
- 1/4 cup softened cream cheese (full-fat)
- 2-3 oz smoked salmon, thinly sliced
- 1/4 cup chopped cucumber
- 1/4 cup chopped red onion
- Fresh dill, for garnish (optional)

Directions:
1. Spread the cream cheese evenly on the romaine lettuce leaves.
2. Layer the smoked salmon, cucumber, and red onion on top of the cream cheese.

3. Roll up the lettuce leaves tightly and enjoy your low-carb and protein-packed wrap. You can optionally heat the wraps in a skillet for a few minutes for a warmer texture.

4. Sprinkle with fresh dill for an extra flavor boost (optional).

Nutritional Values per Serving (approx.):
Calories: 350 | Carbs: 2g | Fat: 30g |
Fiber: 2g | Protein: 20g | Sugar: 1g

Sausage Casserole

Preparation Time: 15 minutes
Cooking Time: 45 minutes
Servings: 4-6

Ingredients:
- 1 pound ground sausage (Italian, chorizo, or your favorite)
- 1 medium onion, chopped
- 2 cloves garlic, minced
- 1 (28 oz) can diced, undrained tomatoes
- 1 (15 oz) can, rinsed and drained cannellini beans
- 1 cup chicken broth
- 1/2 cup chopped bell pepper (any color)
- 1/2 cup chopped spinach
- 1/4 cup chopped fresh parsley
- 1 teaspoon dried oregano
- 1/2 teaspoon salt
- 1/4 teaspoon black pepper
- 1 cup shredded mozzarella cheese

Directions:
1. Preheat oven to 375°F (190°C).

2. Brown the ground sausage in a large skillet over medium heat. Drain any excess fat.

3. Add the onion and garlic to the pan and cook until softened, about 5 minutes.

4. Stir in the diced tomatoes, cannellini beans, chicken broth, bell pepper, spinach, parsley, oregano, salt, and pepper.

5. After bringing to a simmer, cook for five minutes.

6. Transfer the mixture to a baking dish. Top with shredded mozzarella cheese and bake for 25-30 minutes, or until bubbly and cheese is melted.

7. Enjoy this hearty and flavorful casserole with crusty bread or a side salad.

Nutritional Values per Serving (approx.):
Calories: 450 | Carbs: 30g | Fat: 25g |
Fiber: 5g | Protein: 30g | Sugar: 5g

Black Bean Vegan Wraps

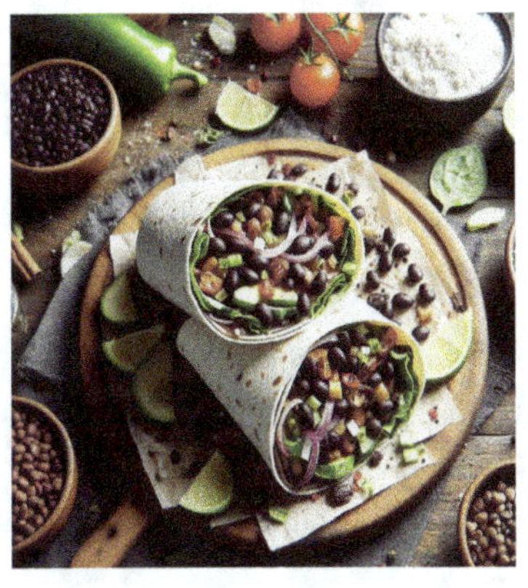

Preparation Time: 15 minutes
Cooking Time: 10 minutes (optional)
Serving: 2

Ingredients:
- 2 whole wheat tortillas
- 1 (15 oz) can, rinsed and drained black beans
- 1/2 cup cooked brown rice or quinoa
- 1/4 cup chopped red onion
- 1/4 cup chopped red bell pepper
- 1/4 cup chopped fresh cilantro
- 1/4 cup salsa
- 1/2 lime, juiced
- 1/4 teaspoon ground cumin
- Salt and pepper to taste

Directions:
1. Heat the black beans in a skillet over medium heat until warmed through (optional).

2. In a bowl, combine the black beans, brown rice or quinoa, red onion, bell pepper, cilantro, salsa, lime juice, cumin, salt, and pepper. Mix well.

3. Spread the filling evenly on the tortillas.

4. Roll up tightly and enjoy your delicious and nutritious vegan wraps.

Nutritional Values per Serving (approx.):
Calories: 350 | Carbs: 37g | Fat: 5g |
Fiber: 8g | Protein: 20g | Sugar: 5g

Cajun Pork Sliders

Preparation Time: 15 minutes
Marinating Time: 30 minutes (optional)
Cooking Time: 10 minutes (grilling)
Servings: 4

Ingredients:
Pork:
- 1 pound boneless, skinless pork shoulder or loin, thinly sliced
- 1/4 cup olive oil
- 2 tablespoons brown sugar
- 1 tablespoon Cajun seasoning
- 1/2 teaspoon salt
- 1/4 teaspoon black pepper

Sliders:
- 4 mini hamburger buns
- Cajun mayo (optional)
- Coleslaw (optional)
- Pickled onions or jalapenos (optional)

Directions:
1. Combine olive oil, brown sugar, Cajun seasoning, salt, and pepper in a bowl. Toss the pork slices with

the marinade and refrigerate for at least 30 minutes for deeper flavor.

2. Prepare your grill or grill pan for medium-high heat.

3. Grill the pork slices for 3-4 minutes per side, or until cooked through.

4. Toast the hamburger buns if desired.

5. Spread with Cajun mayo (optional) and top with grilled pork slices, coleslaw (optional), and pickled onions or jalapenos (optional).

6. Enjoy the spicy and flavorful pork sliders!

Nutritional Values per Serving (approx.):
Calories: 350 | Carbs: 29g | Fat: 20g |
Fiber: 1g | Protein: 30g | Sugar: 5g

Keto Spring Frittata

Preparation Time: 10 minutes
Cooking Time: 20 minutes
Servings: 4

Ingredients:
- 1 tablespoon olive oil
- 1/2 onion, chopped
- 2 cloves garlic, minced
- 1 bell pepper (any color), chopped
- 4 ounces asparagus, chopped
- 8 ounces spinach, chopped
- 8 eggs, beaten
- 1/2 cup shredded cheddar cheese
- 1/4 cup crumbled feta cheese
- Salt and pepper to taste

Directions:
1. Preheat oven to 375°F (190°C).
2. Over medium heat, warm up the olive oil in a big oven-proof skillet. Add the onion, garlic, bell pepper, and asparagus, and cook until softened, about 5 minutes.
3. Cook for a further minute after adding the spinach. Add the whisked eggs and season with

pepper and salt. Cook until the eggs are almost set around the edges.

4. Sprinkle the cheddar cheese and feta cheese over the top of the frittata. Transfer the skillet to the oven and bake for 10-15 minutes, or until the eggs are completely set and the cheese is melted.

5. Cut the frittata into wedges and enjoy a high-protein and low-carb spring-inspired dish.

Nutritional Values per Serving (approx.):
Calories: 350 | Carbs: 1g | Fat: 25g |
Fiber: 1g | Protein: 25g | Sugar: 1g

Low Carb Cauliflower Salad and Shrimp

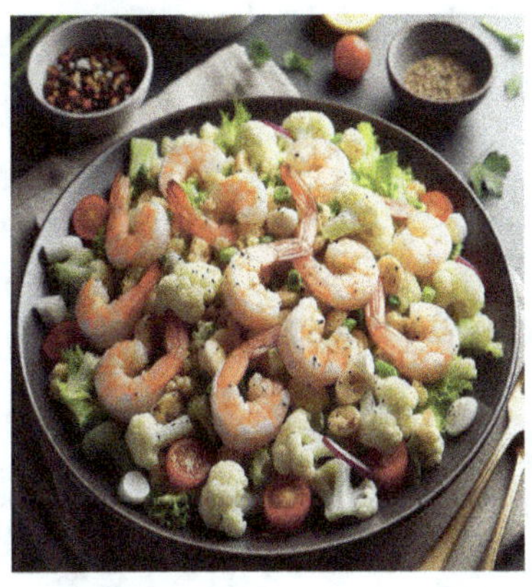

Ingredients:
Salad:
- 1 head cauliflower, grated
- 1/4 cup chopped cucumber
- 1/4 cup chopped red onion
- 1/4 cup chopped fresh parsley
- 2 tablespoons olive oil
- 1 tablespoon apple cider vinegar
- 1/2 teaspoon lemon juice
- Salt and pepper to taste

Shrimp:
- 8 large shrimp, peeled and deveined
- 1 tablespoon olive oil
- 1/2 teaspoon Cajun seasoning

- 1/4 teaspoon garlic powder

Directions:

1. In a large bowl, combine grated cauliflower, cucumber, red onion, and parsley.

2. In a separate smaller bowl, whisk together olive oil, apple cider vinegar, lemon juice, salt, and pepper.

3. Drizzle the salad with the dressing and toss to mix.

4. Heat olive oil in a skillet over medium-high heat. Season the shrimp with Cajun seasoning and garlic powder.

5. Sauté for 3-4 minutes per side, or until cooked through and pink.

6. Top the salad with the cooked shrimp and enjoy a refreshing and protein-packed low-carb dish.

Nutritional Values per Serving (approx.):
Calories: 250 | Carbs: 3g | Fat: 15g |
Fiber: 2g | Protein: 25g | Sugar: 2g

Chapter 7: Desserts/Snacks

Keto Chocolate Mousse
Butterscotch Pumpkin Cream Muffin Bars
Cheese and Veggie Sticks
Chocolate Avocado Mousse
Roasted Chickpeas
Air-Popped Popcorn
Almond Florentine Cookies
Apple Slices with Nut Butter
Muscle Mug Cake
Greek Yogurt with Berries

Keto Chocolate Mousse

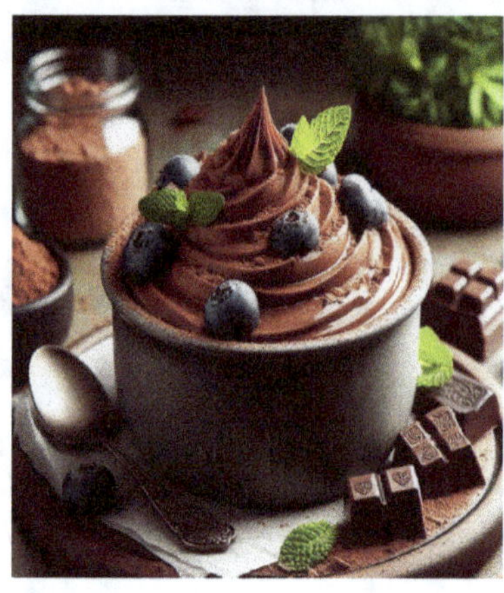

Preparation Time: 10 minutes
Chilling Time: 2 hours
Servings: 4

Ingredients:
- 12 ounces heavy cream
- 1/2 cup dark chocolate, finely chopped
- 1/4 cup granulated erythritol or other keto-friendly sweetener
- 3 large eggs, separated
- 1/2 teaspoon vanilla extract
- Pinch of salt

Directions:
1. In a saucepan, heat the heavy cream over medium heat until simmering.

2. Remove from heat and stir in the chopped chocolate until melted and smooth. Let cool slightly.

3. In a separate bowl, whisk together the egg yolks and sweetener until thick and pale yellow.

4. In another bowl, whip the egg whites and salt to stiff peaks.

5. Gently fold the cooled chocolate mixture into the yolk mixture. Next, gently fold in the whipped egg whites. Finally, stir in the vanilla extract.

6. Divide the mousse into serving dishes and refrigerate for at least 2 hours to set. Enjoy a rich and decadent keto dessert without the guilt.

Nutritional Values per Serving (approx.):
Calories: 350 | Carbs: 1g | Fat: 30g |
Fiber: 1g | Protein: 7g | Sugar: 1g

Butterscotch Pumpkin Cream Muffin Bars

Preparation Time: 15 minutes
Baking Time: 30-35 minutes
Servings: 12

Ingredients:
Dry Ingredients:
- 1 1/2 cups all-purpose flour
- 1/2 cup brown sugar, packed
- 1/2 teaspoon baking powder
- 1/2 teaspoon baking soda
- 1/4 teaspoon salt
- 1/4 teaspoon ground cinnamon
- 1/4 teaspoon ground nutmeg

Wet Ingredients:
- 1/2 cup pumpkin puree
- 1/4 cup melted butter
- 1/4 cup brown sugar, packed
- 1 egg
- 1 teaspoon vanilla extract
- 1/2 cup buttermilk
- Topping:
- 1/2 cup brown sugar, packed
- 1/4 cup butter, softened
- 1/4 cup chopped pecans (optional)

Directions:

1. Preheat oven to 350°F (175°C).Put parchment paper into a 9 × 13-inch baking pan.

2. In a large bowl, whisk together flour, brown sugar, baking powder, baking soda, salt, cinnamon, and nutmeg.

3. In another bowl, whisk together pumpkin puree, melted butter, brown sugar, egg, vanilla extract, and buttermilk.

4. Stir the wet ingredients into the dry ingredients until just combined. Transfer the batter into the ready pan and spread it uniformly.

5. In a small bowl, mix together the brown sugar and softened butter until crumbly. Stir in the chopped pecans (optional). Evenly distribute the topping over the batter.

6. Bake the bars for thirty to thirty-five minutes, or until a toothpick inserted in the middle comes out clean.

7. Let the bars cool in the pan for at least 30 minutes before cutting and serving.

Nutritional Values per Serving (approx.):
Calories: 250 | Carbs: 27g | Fat: 12g |
Fiber: 3g | Protein: 4g | Sugar: 15g

Cheese and Veggie Sticks

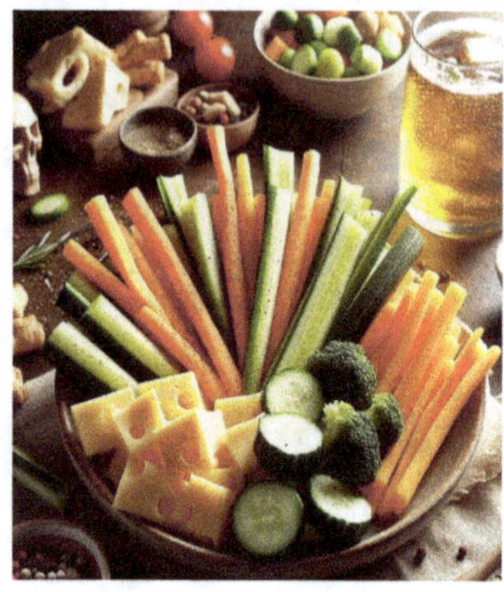

Preparation Time: 5 minutes
Cooking Time: None
Servings: Varies (depending on how much you make)

Ingredients:
- **Variety of cheeses (choose your favorites): cheddar, gouda, mozzarella, swiss, etc.**
- **Variety of vegetables (cut into sticks): carrots, cucumbers, bell peppers, celery, broccoli florets, cherry tomatoes, etc.**
- **Optional accompaniments: hummus, ranch dressing, pesto, olives, nuts, etc.**

Directions:
1. Cut them into sticks or bite-sized pieces, making sure they are easy to hold.

2. Choose your preferred sizes and shapes for easy dipping.

3. Place the cheese and vegetables on a platter or individual plates.

4. Add any desired accompaniments for extra flavor and variety. Enjoy this simple and nutritious snack!

Nutritional Values per Serving (1 cup vegetables + 1 oz cheese):
Calories: 200 | Carbs: 7g | Fat: 10g | Fiber: 3g | Protein: 10g | Sugar: 5g

---

Chocolate Avocado Mousse

Preparation Time: 10 minutes
Chilling Time: 30 minutes (optional)
Servings: 2-3

Ingredients:
- 1 ripe avocado, peeled and pitted
- 1/4 cup unsweetened cocoa powder
- 2 tablespoons honey or maple syrup (or other sweetener of choice)
- 1/4 cup milk (dairy or plant-based)
- 1/4 teaspoon vanilla extract
- Pinch of salt

Directions:
1. In a powerful blender, combine all ingredients and blend until smooth and creamy. Periodically, you might need to pause and scrape down the sides.
2. Taste the mousse and adjust sweetness or other flavors as desired.
3. For a colder and firmer texture, you can chill the mousse in the refrigerator for at least 30 minutes before serving.

4. Divide the mousse into bowls and top with your favorite garnishes like shaved chocolate, berries, or chopped nuts.

Nutritional Values per Serving (approx.):
Calories: 250 | Carbs: 11g | Fat: 20g |
Fiber: 4g | Protein: 4g | Sugar: 10g

Roasted Chickpeas

Prep Time: 10 minutes | Cooking Time: 30-40 minutes | Servings: 2-3

Ingredients:
- 1 (15 oz) can chickpeas, drained and rinsed
- 1 tablespoon olive oil
- 1/2 teaspoon spice blend of your choice (e.g., paprika, cumin, chili powder, garlic powder, etc.)
- Salt and pepper to taste

Directions:
1. Preheat oven to 400°F (200°C).
2. In a bowl, combine chickpeas, olive oil, spices, salt, and pepper. Toss to coat evenly.
3. Spread the chickpeas on a baking sheet in a single layer.
4. Roast for 30-40 minutes, stirring occasionally, until crispy and golden brown.
5. Taste and adjust seasonings if needed. Serve warm as a snack or as part of a salad or bowl.

Nutritional Values per Serving (approx.):
Calories: 200 | Carbs: 10g | Fat: 5g |
Fiber: 10g | Protein: 8g | Sugar: 2g

Air-Popped Popcorn

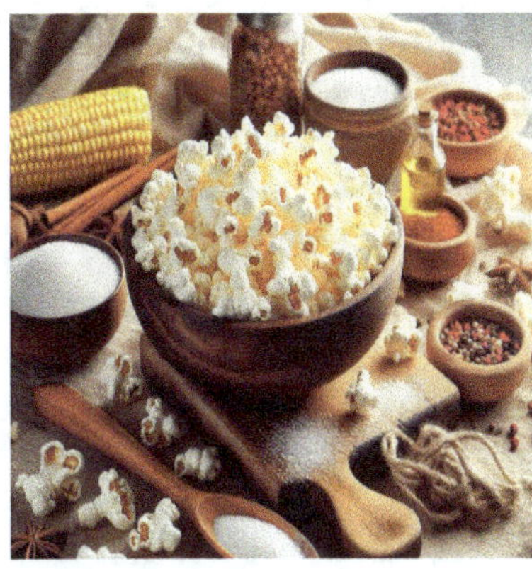

Preparation Time: 5 minutes
Cooking Time: 3-5 minutes
Servings: 3 cups (approximately)

Ingredients:
- 1/4 cup popcorn kernels
- Cooking oil spray (optional, only for stovetop method)
- Salt and spices to taste (optional)

Directions:
1. If using an air popper, simply add the kernels and turn it on. Enjoy fluffy and healthy popcorn without added oil.
2. If using a pot or popcorn maker, heat a thin layer of oil (around 1 tablespoon) until shimmering.
3. Add the popcorn kernels in a single layer, cover loosely, and remove from heat briefly.

4. Listen for the popping sound and return the pot to heat, shaking occasionally, until the popping slows down significantly.

5. Remove the popcorn from heat, season with salt and spices if desired, and savor this light and healthy snack!

Nutritional Values per Serving (approx.):
Calories: 110 | Carbs: 19g | Fat: 1g |
Fiber: 6g | Protein: 3g | Sugar: 1g

Almond Florentine Cookies

Preparation Time: 15 minutes
Baking Time: 10-12 minutes
Servings: 20-24 cookies

Ingredients:
- 1 cup sliced almonds
- 1/3 cup granulated sugar
- 1/3 cup honey
- 1/4 cup butter
- 1/4 cup chopped dark chocolate
- 1/4 teaspoon sea salt

Directions:
1. Preheat oven to 350°F (175°C). Use parchment paper to line a baking sheet.
2. Spread the almonds on a baking sheet and toast in the oven for 5-7 minutes, stirring occasionally, until golden brown.
3. In a saucepan over medium heat, combine sugar and honey. Bring to a simmer and cook, stirring from time to time, until the sugar is completely dissolved.

4. Remove from heat and stir in butter until melted. Add the chopped chocolate and let sit for 1 minute to melt.

5. Pour the caramel mixture over the toasted almonds and stir to coat evenly.

6. Using a teaspoon, drop small mounds of the mixture onto the prepared baking sheet. Bake for 10-12 minutes, or until golden brown and bubbly.

7. Let the cookies cool completely on the baking sheet before sprinkling with sea salt. Enjoy these chewy and decadent cookies with a hint of almond and chocolate!

Nutritional Values per Serving (approx.):
Calories: 100 | Carbs: 11g | Fat: 5g |
Fiber: 1g | Protein: 1g | Sugar: 8g

Apple Slices with Nut Butter

Preparation Time: 5 minutes | Servings: 1-2

Ingredients:
- 1 apple, cored and sliced
- 2-3 tablespoons nut butter of your choice (e.g., peanut, almond, cashew)
- Optional toppings: cinnamon, honey, chia seeds, granola

Directions:
1. Choose a crisp and juicy apple like a Gala, Honeycrisp, or Fuji. Wash and core it, then slice into thin wedges or sticks.
2. Spread your preferred nut butter on the apple slices to your desired thickness.
3. Feel free to sprinkle with cinnamon, honey, chia seeds, or granola for extra flavor and texture.

Nutritional Values per Serving (2 apple slices with 2 tablespoons almond butter):
Calories: 200 | Carbs: 20g | Fat: 8g |
Fiber: 5g | Protein: 5g | Sugar: 10g

Muscle Mug Cake

Prep Time: 5 minutes | Cooking Time: 1-2 minutes (microwave) | Servings: 1

Ingredients:
- 1/4 cup rolled oats
- 1/4 cup scoop protein powder (chocolate, vanilla, or your favorite flavor)
- 1/4 cup unsweetened almond milk
- 1 tablespoon unsweetened applesauce
- 1/2 teaspoon baking powder
- Pinch of salt
- Optional toppings: fresh berries, chopped nuts, nut butter drizzle

Directions:

1. In a microwave-safe mug, combine rolled oats, protein powder, almond milk, applesauce, baking powder, and salt. Stir until well combined.
2. Microwave on high for 1-2 minutes, or until the cake is cooked through and slightly fluffy.
3. Let cool slightly, then top with your preferred toppings and enjoy!

Nutritional Values (approx.):
Calories: 250 | Carbs: 20g | Fat: 5g |
Fiber: 5g | Protein: 20g | Sugar: 5g

Greek Yogurt with Berries

Preparation Time: 5 minutes | Servings: 1

Ingredients:
- 1 cup plain Greek yogurt (low-fat or full-fat, depending on your preference)
- 1/2 cup fresh berries (blueberries, raspberries, strawberries, etc.)
- 1 tablespoon honey or maple syrup (optional)
- 1/4 cup chopped nuts or granola (optional)

Directions:
1. Spoon the Greek yogurt into a bowl or container.
2. Top with your favorite berries.
3. If preferred, drizzle with honey or maple syrup.
4. Sprinkle with chopped nuts or granola for added texture and flavor.
5. Enjoy this refreshing and healthy snack!

Nutritional Values (approx.):
Calories: 200 | Carbs: 17g | Fat: 5g |
Fiber: 3g | Protein: 15g | Sugar: 10g

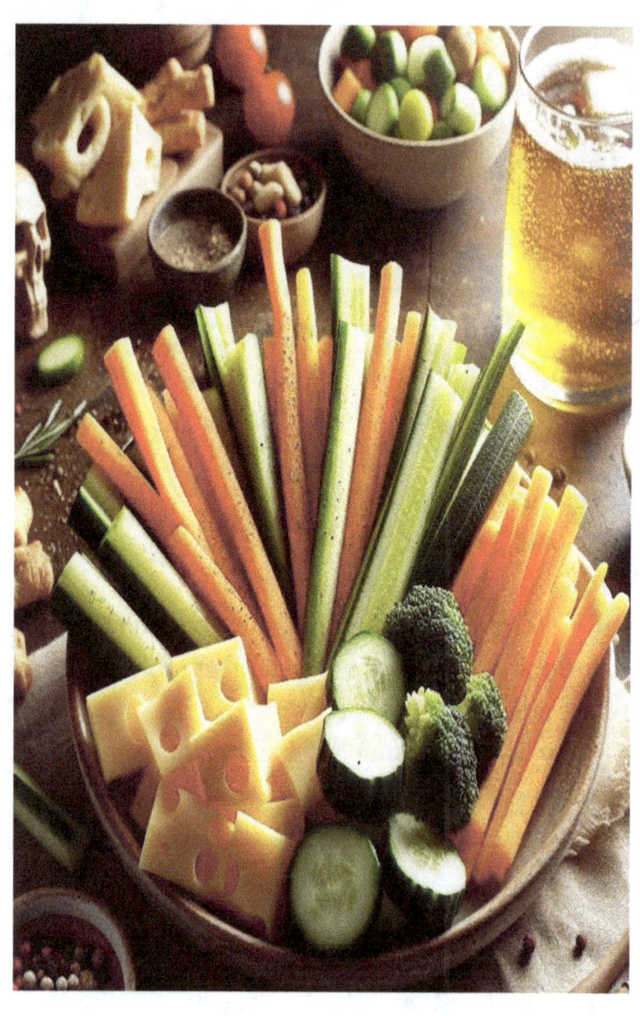

Chapter 8: Smoothie Recipes

Collagen Berry Banana Smoothie
Turmeric Pineapple Smoothie
Minty Matcha Smoothie
Banana and Greens Smoothie
Strawberry Banana Smoothie
Blueberry Hemp Smoothie
Mango and Greens Smoothie
Kale, Apple, and Ginger Smoothie
Tropical Smoothie
Carrot Orange Smoothie

Collagen Berry Banana Smoothie

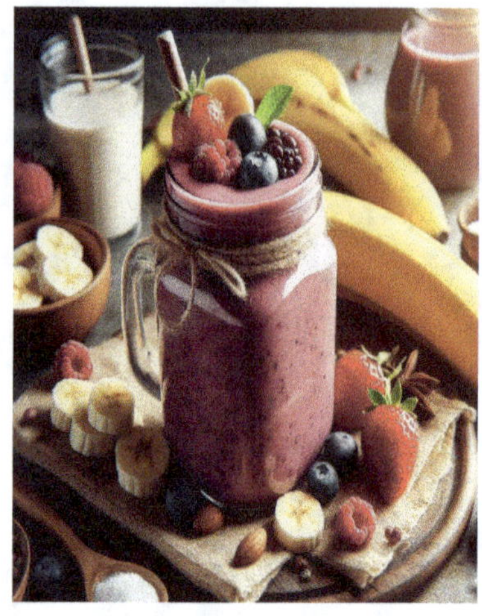

**Preparation Time:
5 minutes
Servings: 1**

Ingredients:
- 1 scoop unflavored collagen powder
- 1 cup frozen mixed berries
- 1 frozen banana
- 1/2 cup unsweetened almond milk (or milk of your choice)
- 1/4 cup Greek yogurt, optional for extra protein
- 1/2 teaspoon vanilla extract (optional)
- Ice cubes (optional, adjust for desired thickness)

Directions:
1. Blend all ingredients until smooth and creamy.
2. Enjoy immediately!

Nutritional Values per Serving (approx.):
Calories: 250 | Carbs: 22g | Fat: 5-10g |
Fiber: 8g | Protein: 25g | Sugar: 10

Turmeric Pineapple Smoothie

Preparation Time: 5 minutes | Servings: 1

Ingredients:
- 1/2 teaspoon ground turmeric
- 1/2 cup frozen pineapple chunks
- 1/2 ripe banana
- 1/2 cup unsweetened coconut water (or milk of your choice)
- 1/4 cup Greek yogurt, optional for extra protein
- 1 tablespoon chopped fresh ginger (optional)
- 1/4 teaspoon ground cinnamon (optional)
- Ice cubes (optional, adjust for desired thickness)

Directions:
1. Blend all ingredients until smooth and creamy.
2. Enjoy immediately!

Nutritional Values per Serving (approx.):
Calories: 200 | Carbs: 25g | Fat: 5g |
Fiber: 7g | Protein: 7g | Sugar: 15g

Minty Matcha Smoothie

Preparation Time: 5 minutes | Servings: 1

Ingredients:
- 1/2 teaspoon matcha powder
- 1/2 cup fresh spinach leaves
- 1/2 frozen banana
- 1 cup unsweetened almond milk (or any other milk of your choice)
- 1/4 cup Greek yogurt, optional for extra protein
- 1/4 teaspoon peppermint extract
- Ice cubes (optional, adjust for desired thickness)

Directions:
1. Blend all ingredients until smooth and creamy.
2. Enjoy immediately!

Nutritional Values per Serving (approx.):
**Calories: 150 | Carbs: 20 | Fat: 2g |
Fiber: 7g | Protein: 10g | Sugar: 5g**

Banana and Greens Smoothie

Preparation Time: 5 minutes | Servings: 1

Ingredients:
- 1 frozen banana
- 1/2 cup leafy greens (spinach, kale, etc.)
- 1/2 cup water (or milk of your choice)
- 1/2 cup yogurt (plain or Greek, optional for added protein)
- 1 scoop protein powder (optional)
- 1/2 teaspoon almond butter (optional for creaminess)
- Pinch of cinnamon (optional)
- Ice cubes (optional, adjust for desired thickness)

Directions:
1. Blend all ingredients until smooth and creamy.
2. Enjoy immediately!

Nutritional Values per Serving (approx.):
Calories: 250 | Carbs: 25g | Fat: 5g |
Fiber: 8g | Protein: 20g | Sugar: 10g

Strawberry Banana Smoothie

Preparation Time: 5 minutes | Servings: 1

Ingredients:
- 1 frozen banana
- 1 cup frozen strawberries
- 1/2 cup milk of your choice
- 1/4 cup yogurt (plain or Greek, optional)
- 1/2 teaspoon maple syrup or honey (optional)
- Pinch of vanilla extract (optional)
- Ice cubes (optional, adjust for desired thickness)

Directions:
1. Blend all ingredients until smooth and creamy.
2. Enjoy immediately!

Nutritional Values per Serving (approx.):
Calories: 200 | Carbs: 30g | Fat: 10g |
Fiber: 7g | Protein: 8g | Sugar: 15g

Blueberry Hemp Smoothie

Preparation Time: 5 minutes | Servings: 1

Ingredients:
- 1/2 cup frozen blueberries
- 1/2 cup yogurt (plain or Greek)
- 1/2 cup milk of your choice
- 1 tablespoon hemp seeds
- 1/2 teaspoon maple syrup or honey (optional)
- Pinch of cinnamon (optional)
- Ice cubes (optional, adjust for desired thickness)

Directions:
1. Blend all ingredients until smooth and creamy.
2. Enjoy immediately!

Nutritional Values per Serving (approx.):
Calories: 250 | Carbs: 35g | Fat: 10g |
Fiber: 7g | Protein: 15g | Sugar: 15g

Mango and Greens Smoothie

Preparation Time: 5 minutes | Servings: 1

Ingredients:
- 1/2 cup frozen mango chunks
- 1/2 cup leafy greens (spinach, kale, etc.)
- 1/2 cup water (or milk of your choice)
- 1/4 cup yogurt (plain or Greek, optional)
- 1 scoop protein powder (optional)
- Pinch of ginger (optional)
- Ice cubes (optional, adjust for desired thickness)

Directions:
1. Blend all ingredients until smooth and creamy.
2. Enjoy immediately!

Nutritional Values per Serving (approx.):
Calories: 300 | Carbs: 30g | Fat: 5g |
Fiber: 8g | Protein: 20g | Sugar: 15g

Kale, Apple, and Ginger Smoothie

Preparation Time: 5 minutes | Servings: 1

Ingredients:
- 1/2 cup finely chopped baby spinach or kale
- 1/2 apple, cored and chopped
- 1/2 inch fresh ginger, peeled and grated
- 1 banana, frozen or fresh
- 1/2 cup unsweetened almond milk (or milk of your choice)
- 1/4 cup Greek yogurt, optional for extra protein
- 1/4 teaspoon ground cinnamon (optional)
- Ice cubes (optional, adjust for desired thickness)

Directions:
1. Blend all ingredients until smooth and creamy.
2. Enjoy immediately!

Nutritional Values per Serving (approx.):
**Calories: 200 | Carbs: 30g | Fat: 5g |
Fiber: 7g | Protein: 7g | Sugar: 10g**

Tropical Smoothie

Preparation Time: 5 minutes | Servings: 1

Ingredients:
- 1/2 cup frozen mango chunks
- 1/2 cup frozen pineapple chunks
- 1/2 banana, frozen or fresh
- 1/2 cup unsweetened coconut water (or milk of your choice)
- 1/4 cup Greek yogurt, optional for extra protein
- 1/4 teaspoon ground turmeric (optional, for vibrant color)
- Ice cubes (optional, adjust for desired thickness)

Directions:
1. Blend all ingredients until smooth and creamy.
2. Enjoy immediately!

Nutritional Values per Serving (approx.):
Calories: 250 | Carbs: 40g | Fat: 7g |
Fiber: 7g | Protein: 8g | Sugar: 20g

Carrot Orange Smoothie

Preparation Time: 5 minutes | Servings: 1

Ingredients:
- 1/2 cup chopped carrots
- 1/2 orange, peeled and segmented
- 1/2 apple, cored and chopped
- 1/2 banana, frozen or fresh
- 1/2 cup unsweetened almond milk (or milk of your choice)
- 1/4 teaspoon ground cinnamon (optional)
- 1/4 teaspoon ground ginger (optional)
- Ice cubes (optional, adjust for desired thickness)

Directions:
1. Blend all ingredients until smooth and creamy.
2. Enjoy immediately!

Nutritional Values per Serving (approx.):
Calories: 200 | Carbs: 30g | Fat: 5g |
Fiber: 5g | Protein: 10g | Sugar: 15g

Chapter 9: Exercise and Lifestyle Practices: Dancing with Intermittent Fasting

Welcome back, fabulous fasting fanatics! We've explored the diverse flavors of intermittent fasting methods and crafted meal plans to keep your tummies happy. Now, it's time to add movement and mindful habits to the mix, transforming your entire well-being with a harmonious blend of body and soul.

Exercise: Your Intermittent Fasting Ally:

Just like adding spices enhances the taste of a dish, regular physical activity amplifies the benefits of intermittent fasting. Think of it as a dynamic duo, working together to boost your energy, strength, and overall health.

Gentle Yet Effective Movement:

Gentle, low-impact exercises are perfect for women over 60, especially while adjusting to intermittent fasting. Here are some delightful options to get you moving:

- **Morning walks**: Embrace the sunrise with a brisk walk, soaking in the fresh air and boosting your mood.
- **Water workouts**: Gentle water walking or aqua aerobics offer low-impact strength training and cardiovascular benefits without joint stress.
- **Yoga**: Flow through calming yoga poses to improve flexibility, reduce stress, and enhance core strength.
- **Pilates**: This mindful exercise practice tones muscles, improves balance, and strengthens your core, promoting better posture and stability.

Remember: Start slow, listen to your body, and gradually increase intensity and duration as you progress. Aim for at least 30 minutes of moderate-intensity exercise most days of the week; consistency is essential.

Strength Training: Your Inner Warrior Awaits:

Building muscle mass is crucial, especially after 60, to combat age-related muscle loss and maintain strong bones. Don't be intimidated by weights! Incorporate light strength training using dumbbells, resistance bands, or even your own body weight.

Lifestyle Practices for a Holistic Harmony

Beyond exercise, several lifestyle practices can empower your intermittent fasting journey and enhance your overall well-being:

- **Stress Management**: Chronic stress can hinder your progress. Practice relaxation techniques like meditation, deep breathing, or spending time in nature to keep stress at bay.
- **Quality Sleep**: Aim for 7-8 hours of restful sleep each night. Adequate sleep regulates hormones, promotes recovery, and boosts energy levels.
- **Social Connection**: Surround yourself with supportive loved ones who encourage your healthy choices. Social interaction promotes emotional well-being and provides motivation.
- **Gratitude Practice**: Cultivating an attitude of gratitude can improve your mood, reduce stress, and enhance overall well-being. Start a gratitude journal or simply take time each

day to appreciate the good things in your life.

Remember: Consistency and small, gradual changes are key to sustainable success. Celebrate your progress, be kind to yourself, and enjoy the journey of creating a healthier, happier you.

I hope this chapter resonates with you and inspires you to incorporate movement and mindful practices into your intermittent fasting journey.

14-Day Intermittent Fasting Meal Plan

Day 1:
Breakfast: Hearty Pancakes
Lunch: Salmon and Green Beans
Dinner: Chicken Skewers with Rosemary Buttermilk
Snack: Apple Slices with Nut Butter

Day 2:
Breakfast: Pomegranate Quinoa Porridge
Lunch: Kale and Wild Rice Stir Fry
Dinner: Zucchini Pasta with Pesto Sauce
Snack: Roasted Chickpeas

Day 3:
Breakfast: Greek Yogurt with Berries
Lunch: Steamed Vegetable Pan
Dinner: Veggie Black Bean Burger
Snack: Air-Popped Popcorn

Day 4:
Breakfast: Almond Flour Pancakes
Lunch: Low Carb Stuffed Zucchini and BBQ
Dinner: Sausage Casserole
Snack: Cheese and Veggie Sticks

Day 5:
Breakfast: Tomato and Egg Scramble
Lunch: Black Bean Vegan Wraps
Dinner: Keto Spring Frittata
Snack: Chocolate Avocado Mousse

Day 6:
Breakfast: Pineapple Oatmeal
Lunch: Chicken Breast with Pan Vegetables
Dinner: Keto Wraps with Cream Cheese and Salmon
Snack: Almond Florentine Cookies

Day 7:
Breakfast: Mexican Avocado Salad
Lunch: Toasted and Grilled Pecan Vinaigrette
Dinner: Chili Omelet
Snack: Yogurt Sauce with Chicken Souvlaki

Day 8:

Breakfast: Egg Muffins
Lunch: Sweet Corn Soup
Dinner: Cajun Pork Sliders
Snack: Butterscotch Pumpkin Cream Muffin Bars

Day 9:

Breakfast: Carrot Orange Smoothie
Lunch: Lean Beef Vegetable Soup
Dinner: Avocado Salsa with Grilled Salmon
Snack: Cheese and Veggie Sticks

Day 10:

Breakfast: Waffles with Whipped Cream
Lunch: Zucchini Omelet
Dinner: Flavorful Pumpkin Pie Oatmeal
Snack: Roasted Chickpeas

Day 11:

Breakfast: Minty Matcha Smoothie
Lunch: Kale and Wild Rice Stir Fry
Dinner: Black Bean Vegan Wraps
Snack: Air-Popped Popcorn

Breakfast: Strawberry Banana Smoothie
Lunch: Low Carb Stuffed Zucchini and BBQ
Dinner: Keto Spring Frittata
Snack: Muscle Mug Cake

Breakfast: Blueberry Hemp Smoothie
Lunch: Chicken Breast with Pan Vegetables
Dinner: Avocado Salsa with Grilled Salmon
Snack: Keto Chocolate Mousse

Conclusion

Alright, ladies, we've danced our way through this book, exploring the rhythm of intermittent fasting and how it unlocks a symphony of well-being in your body. You've learned the science, mastered the methods, whipped up some deliciousness in the kitchen, and even swayed with some mindful practices. Now, it's time to drop the mic and step out the door, your confidence radiating like a disco ball in a power outage.

But before you go, let's leave some glitter on the floor, okay? Remember, this isn't a one-shot deal or a fad diet finale. It's a lifestyle remix, a chance to rewrite the melody of your health every day.

Keep these beats going:

- **Celebrate the small wins**: High fives for ditching the afternoon sugar crash! Applause for those extra ten minutes on the treadmill! Every step on this journey deserves a victory dance.
- **Befriend your body**: Ditch the self-criticism and listen to your inner DJ. Craving some avocado? Play that funky beat! Energy lagging? Hit the pause button and catch some zzz's. Your body talks, listen up.
- **Find your groove**: Forget kale smoothies if they make you grimace. Find healthy choices that make you wanna do a happy

dance. Spicy chicken bowls? Salsa classes? You do you, boo.

- **Embrace the tribe**: We all need a cheer squad, ladies. Find your workout buddies, your recipe-sharing pals, your "I hate squats too" support group. Surround yourself with good vibes and keep the party going.

Remember, you're not just rocking a new diet, you're rocking a whole new chapter of your life. It's about feeling strong, energized, and ready to take on the world in sequined leggings and a smile. So, keep the music pumping, keep the body grooving, and keep embracing the power of healthy choices.

This book may be ending, but your health symphony is just getting started. Go forth, conquer your cravings, own your well-being, and show the world what happens when a woman over 60 decides to rewrite the rules and dance to her own tune. You're fabulous, you're fierce, and you're unstoppable. Now go out there and prove it!

Mic drop. Glitter explosion. And one final strut off the stage, knowing you've just created a masterpiece of a life, fueled by the magic of intermittent fasting and the rhythm of your own badass self.

Rock on, queens!

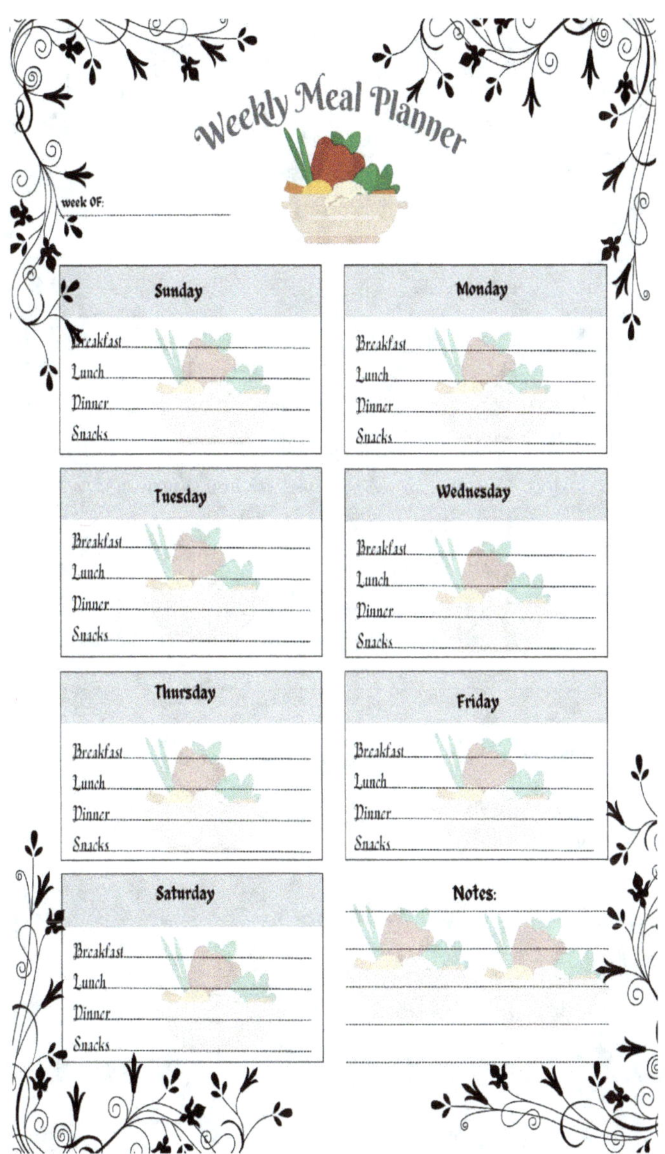

Weekly Meal Planner
week OF:

Sunday
Breakfast
Lunch
Dinner
Snacks

Monday
Breakfast
Lunch
Dinner
Snacks

Tuesday
Breakfast
Lunch
Dinner
Snacks

Wednesday
Breakfast
Lunch
Dinner
Snacks

Thursday
Breakfast
Lunch
Dinner
Snacks

Friday
Breakfast
Lunch
Dinner
Snacks

Saturday
Breakfast
Lunch
Dinner
Snacks

Notes:

Weekly Meal Planner

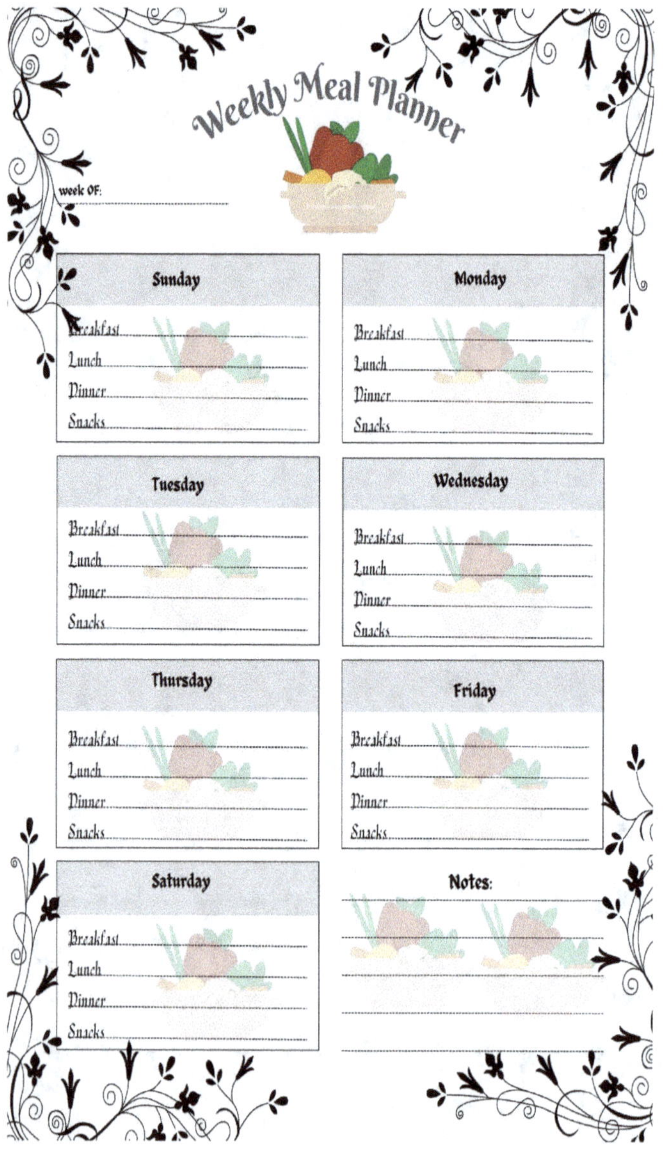

week OF: ______________________

Sunday

Breakfast ....
Lunch ....
Dinner ....
Snacks ....

Monday

Breakfast ....
Lunch ....
Dinner ....
Snacks ....

Tuesday

Breakfast ....
Lunch ....
Dinner ....
Snacks ....

Wednesday

Breakfast ....
Lunch ....
Dinner ....
Snacks ....

Thursday

Breakfast ....
Lunch ....
Dinner ....
Snacks ....

Friday

Breakfast ....
Lunch ....
Dinner ....
Snacks ....

Saturday

Breakfast ....
Lunch ....
Dinner ....
Snacks ....

Notes:

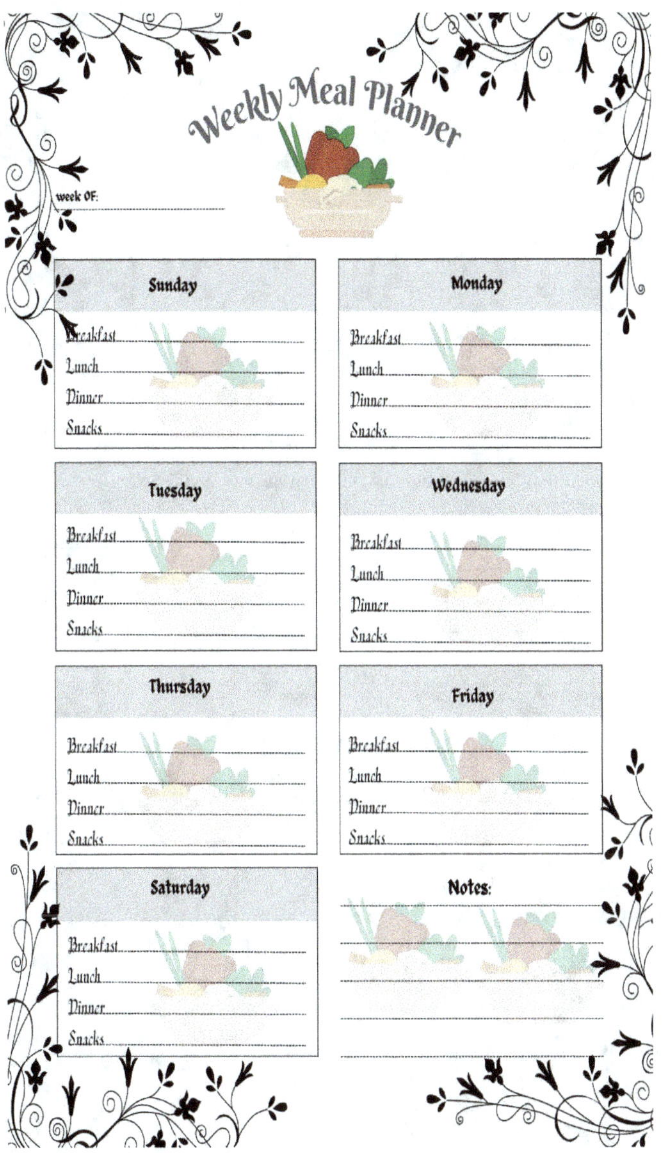

Weekly Meal Planner

week OF:

Sunday
Breakfast
Lunch
Dinner
Snacks

Monday
Breakfast
Lunch
Dinner
Snacks

Tuesday
Breakfast
Lunch
Dinner
Snacks

Wednesday
Breakfast
Lunch
Dinner
Snacks

Thursday
Breakfast
Lunch
Dinner
Snacks

Friday
Breakfast
Lunch
Dinner
Snacks

Saturday
Breakfast
Lunch
Dinner
Snacks

Notes:

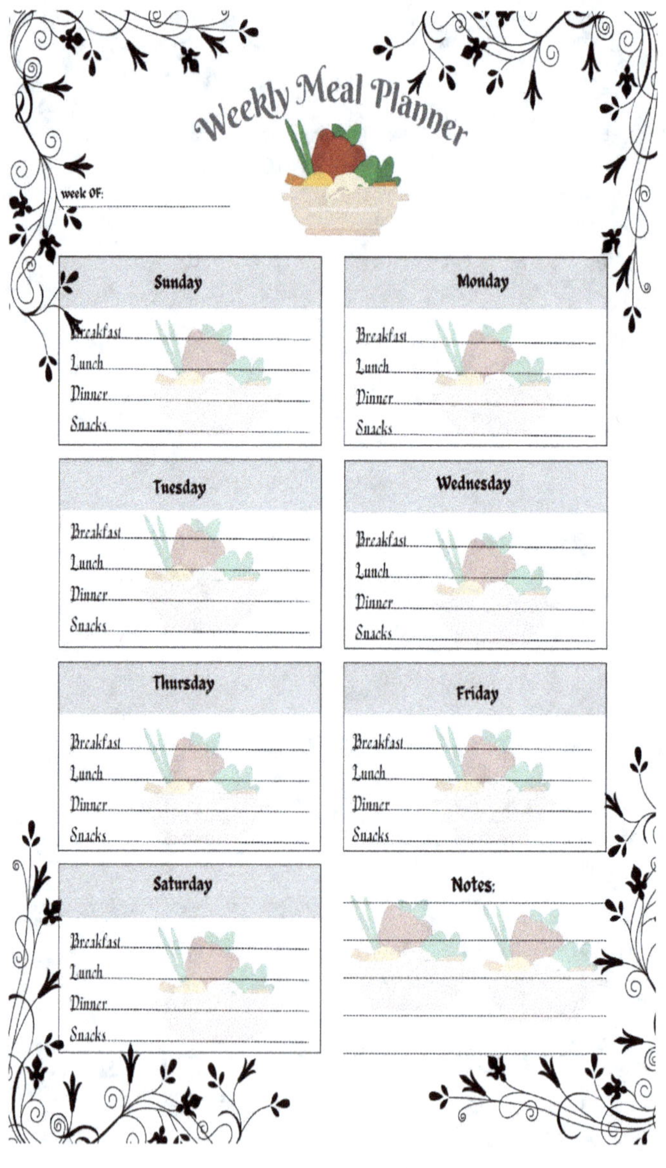

Weekly Meal Planner

week OF:

Sunday
Breakfast
Lunch
Dinner
Snacks

Monday
Breakfast
Lunch
Dinner
Snacks

Tuesday
Breakfast
Lunch
Dinner
Snacks

Wednesday
Breakfast
Lunch
Dinner
Snacks

Thursday
Breakfast
Lunch
Dinner
Snacks

Friday
Breakfast
Lunch
Dinner
Snacks

Saturday
Breakfast
Lunch
Dinner
Snacks

Notes:

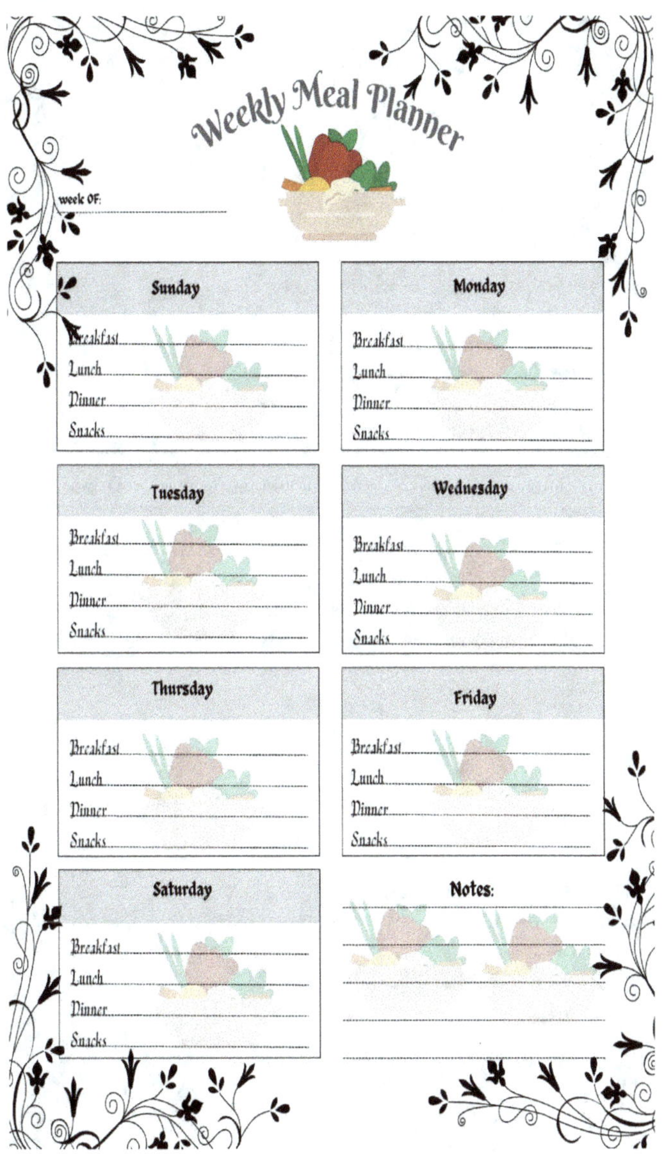

Weekly Meal Planner

week OF:

Sunday
Breakfast
Lunch
Dinner
Snacks

Monday
Breakfast
Lunch
Dinner
Snacks

Tuesday
Breakfast
Lunch
Dinner
Snacks

Wednesday
Breakfast
Lunch
Dinner
Snacks

Thursday
Breakfast
Lunch
Dinner
Snacks

Friday
Breakfast
Lunch
Dinner
Snacks

Saturday
Breakfast
Lunch
Dinner
Snacks

Notes:

Weekly Meal Planner

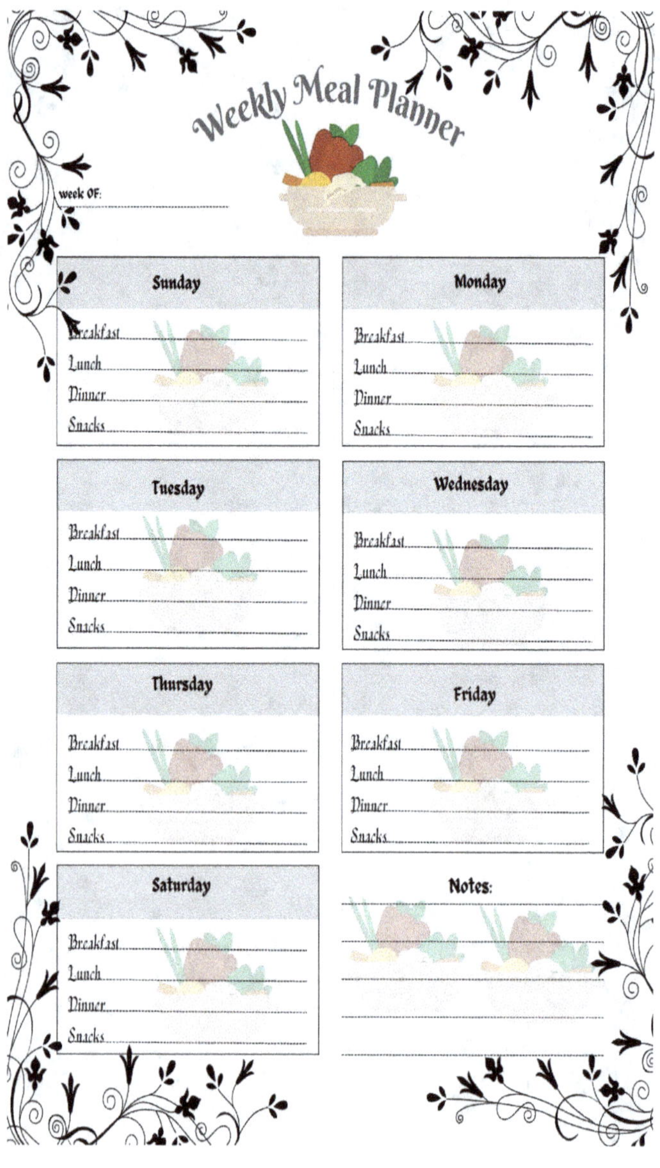

week OF:

Sunday

Breakfast ....
Lunch ....
Dinner ....
Snacks ....

Monday

Breakfast ....
Lunch ....
Dinner ....
Snacks ....

Tuesday

Breakfast ....
Lunch ....
Dinner ....
Snacks ....

Wednesday

Breakfast ....
Lunch ....
Dinner ....
Snacks ....

Thursday

Breakfast ....
Lunch ....
Dinner ....
Snacks ....

Friday

Breakfast ....
Lunch ....
Dinner ....
Snacks ....

Saturday

Breakfast ....
Lunch ....
Dinner ....
Snacks ....

Notes:

Weekly Meal Planner

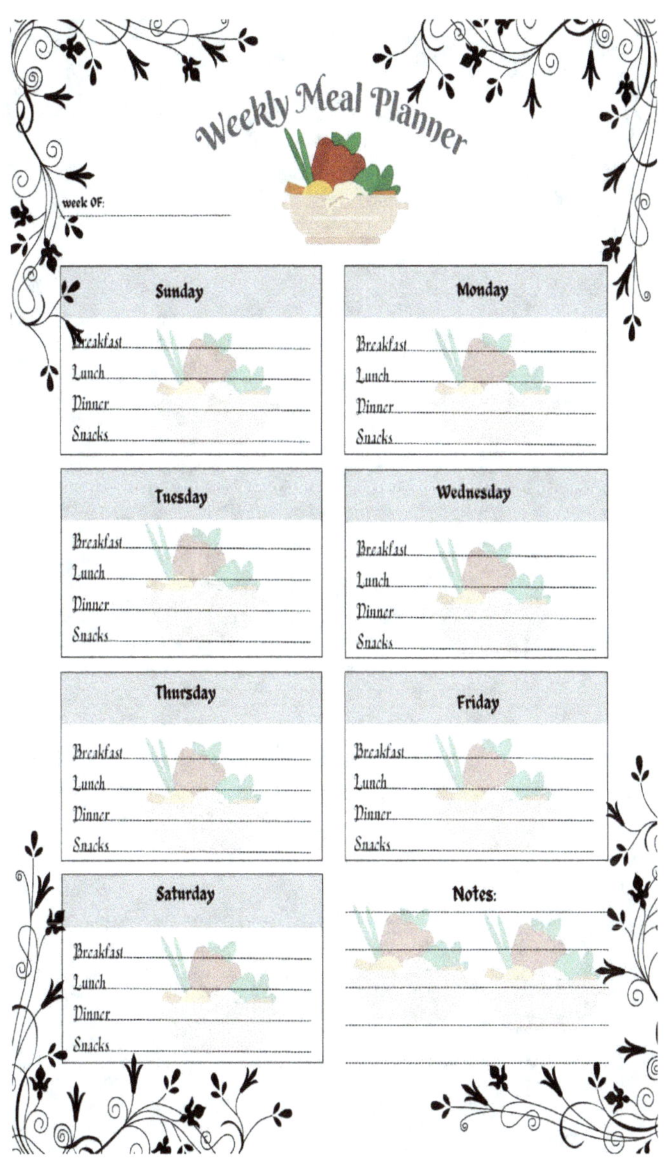

week OF: __________

Sunday

Breakfast ______________
Lunch ______________
Dinner ______________
Snacks ______________

Monday

Breakfast ______________
Lunch ______________
Dinner ______________
Snacks ______________

Tuesday

Breakfast ______________
Lunch ______________
Dinner ______________
Snacks ______________

Wednesday

Breakfast ______________
Lunch ______________
Dinner ______________
Snacks ______________

Thursday

Breakfast ______________
Lunch ______________
Dinner ______________
Snacks ______________

Friday

Breakfast ______________
Lunch ______________
Dinner ______________
Snacks ______________

Saturday

Breakfast ______________
Lunch ______________
Dinner ______________
Snacks ______________

Notes:

____
____
____
____

Weekly Meal Planner

week OF: _______________

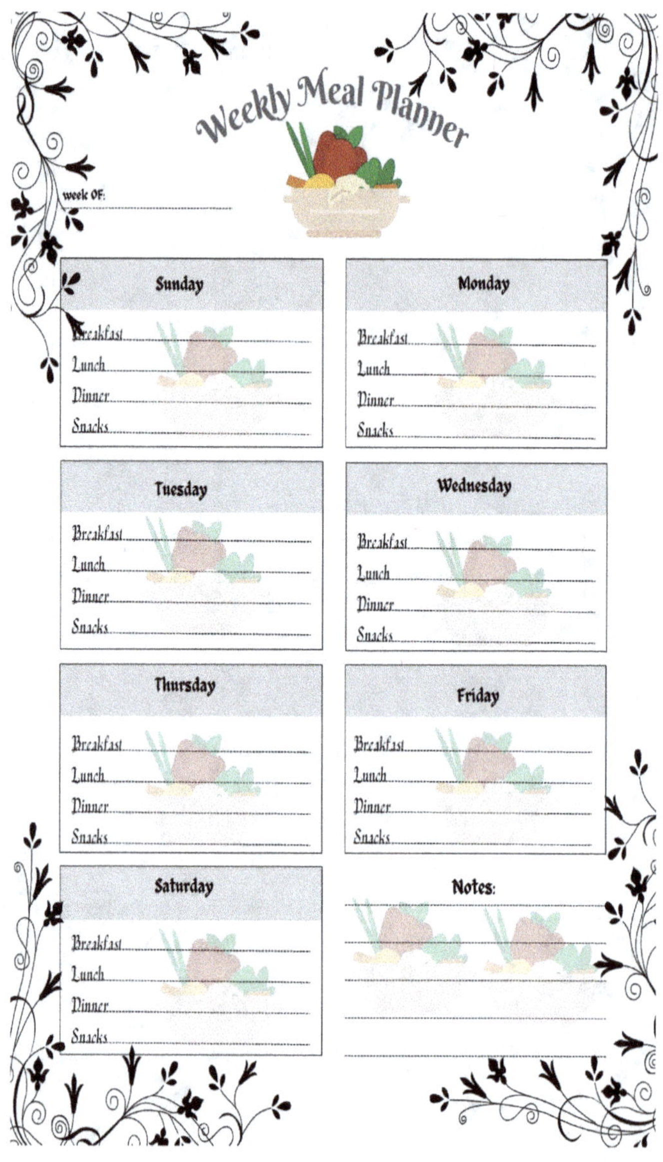

Sunday	Monday
Breakfast	Breakfast
Lunch	Lunch
Dinner	Dinner
Snacks	Snacks

Tuesday	Wednesday
Breakfast	Breakfast
Lunch	Lunch
Dinner	Dinner
Snacks	Snacks

Thursday	Friday
Breakfast	Breakfast
Lunch	Lunch
Dinner	Dinner
Snacks	Snacks

Saturday	Notes:
Breakfast	
Lunch	
Dinner	
Snacks	

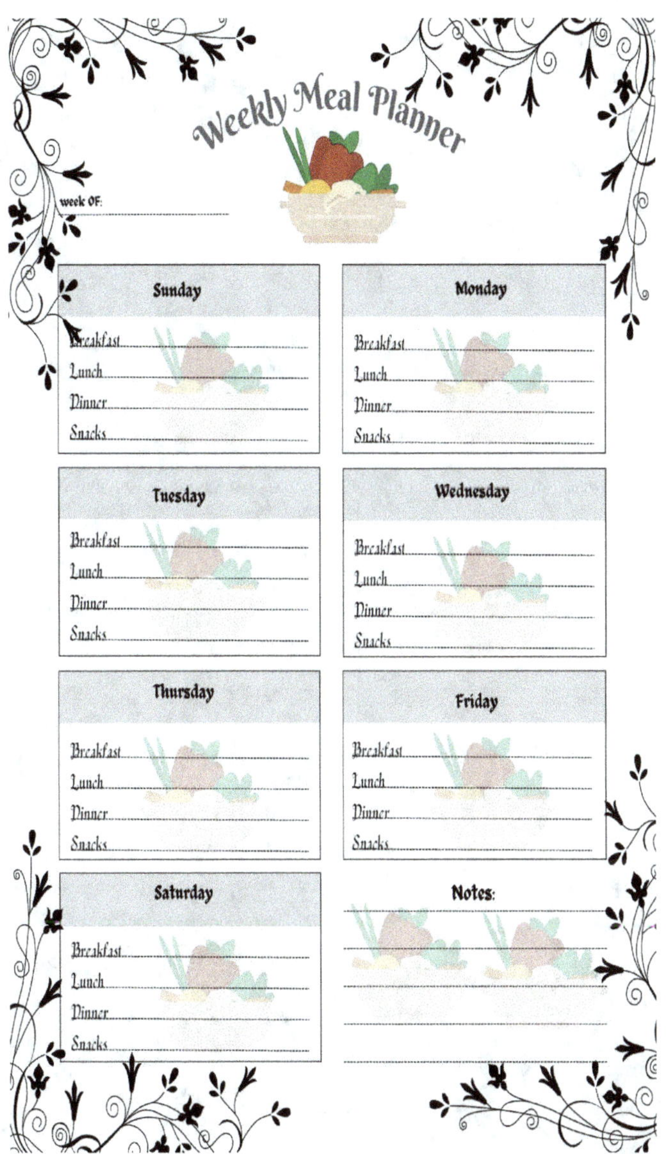

Weekly Meal Planner

week OF:

Sunday
Breakfast
Lunch
Dinner
Snacks

Monday
Breakfast
Lunch
Dinner
Snacks

Tuesday
Breakfast
Lunch
Dinner
Snacks

Wednesday
Breakfast
Lunch
Dinner
Snacks

Thursday
Breakfast
Lunch
Dinner
Snacks

Friday
Breakfast
Lunch
Dinner
Snacks

Saturday
Breakfast
Lunch
Dinner
Snacks

Notes:

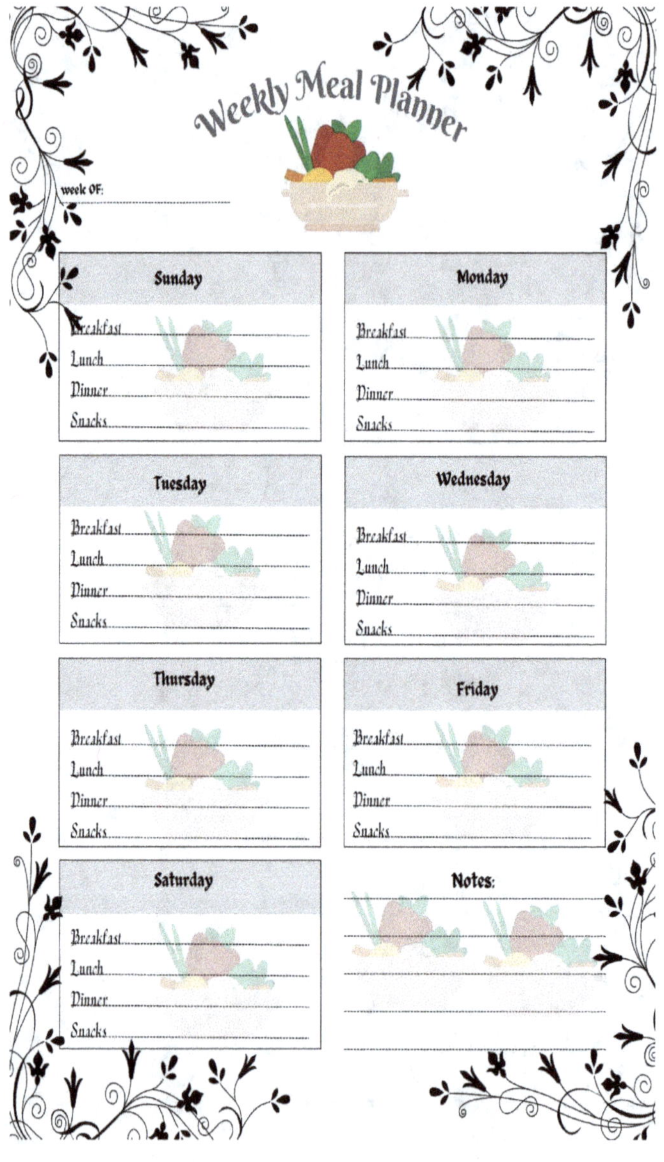

Weekly Meal Planner

week OF:

Sunday
Breakfast
Lunch
Dinner
Snacks

Monday
Breakfast
Lunch
Dinner
Snacks

Tuesday
Breakfast
Lunch
Dinner
Snacks

Wednesday
Breakfast
Lunch
Dinner
Snacks

Thursday
Breakfast
Lunch
Dinner
Snacks

Friday
Breakfast
Lunch
Dinner
Snacks

Saturday
Breakfast
Lunch
Dinner
Snacks

Notes:

Weekly Meal Planner

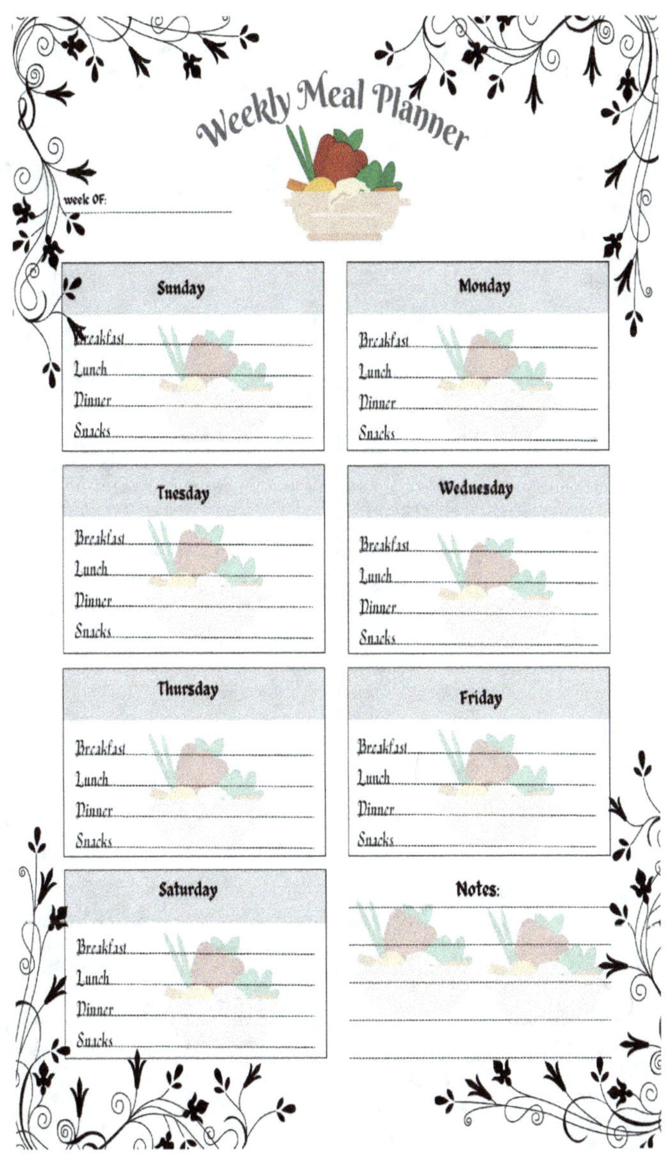

week OF: ....

Sunday

Breakfast ....
Lunch ....
Dinner ....
Snacks ....

Monday

Breakfast ....
Lunch ....
Dinner ....
Snacks ....

Tuesday

Breakfast ....
Lunch ....
Dinner ....
Snacks ....

Wednesday

Breakfast ....
Lunch ....
Dinner ....
Snacks ....

Thursday

Breakfast ....
Lunch ....
Dinner ....
Snacks ....

Friday

Breakfast ....
Lunch ....
Dinner ....
Snacks ....

Saturday

Breakfast ....
Lunch ....
Dinner ....
Snacks ....

Notes:

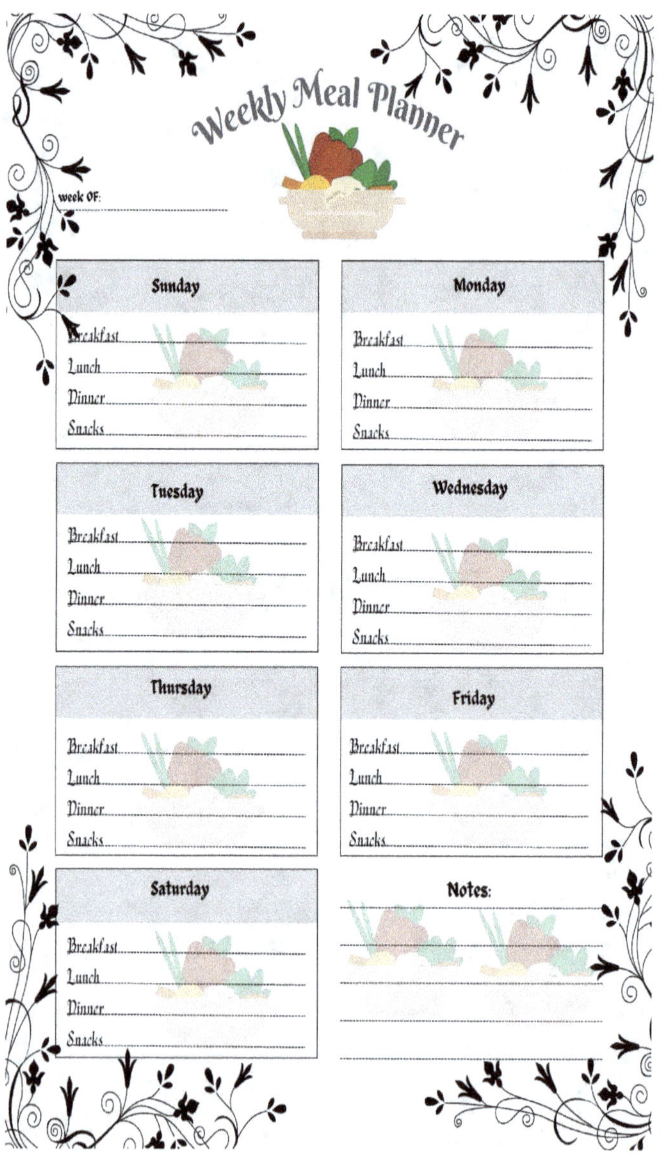

Weekly Meal Planner
week OF:
Sunday
Breakfast
Lunch
Dinner
Snacks
Monday
Breakfast
Lunch
Dinner
Snacks
Tuesday
Breakfast
Lunch
Dinner
Snacks
Wednesday
Breakfast
Lunch
Dinner
Snacks
Thursday
Breakfast
Lunch
Dinner
Snacks
Friday
Breakfast
Lunch
Dinner
Snacks
Saturday
Breakfast
Lunch
Dinner
Snacks
Notes:

Weekly Meal Planner

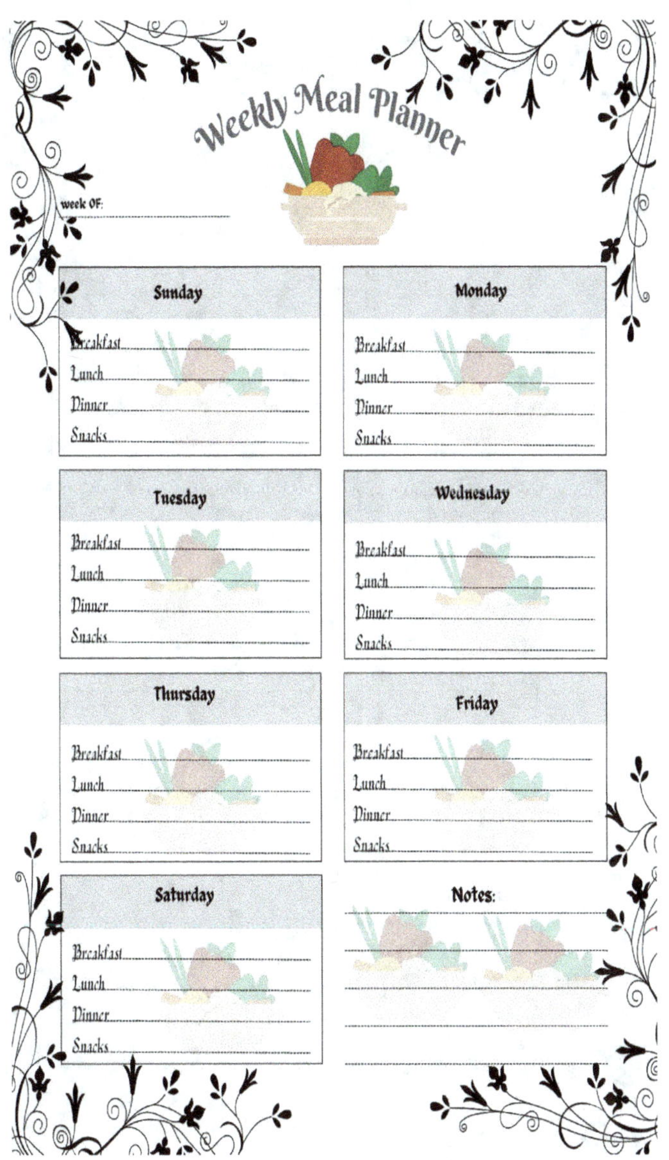

week OF: _______________

Sunday

Breakfast ....
Lunch ....
Dinner ....
Snacks ....

Monday

Breakfast ....
Lunch ....
Dinner ....
Snacks ....

Tuesday

Breakfast ....
Lunch ....
Dinner ....
Snacks ....

Wednesday

Breakfast ....
Lunch ....
Dinner ....
Snacks ....

Thursday

Breakfast ....
Lunch ....
Dinner ....
Snacks ....

Friday

Breakfast ....
Lunch ....
Dinner ....
Snacks ....

Saturday

Breakfast ....
Lunch ....
Dinner ....
Snacks ....

Notes:

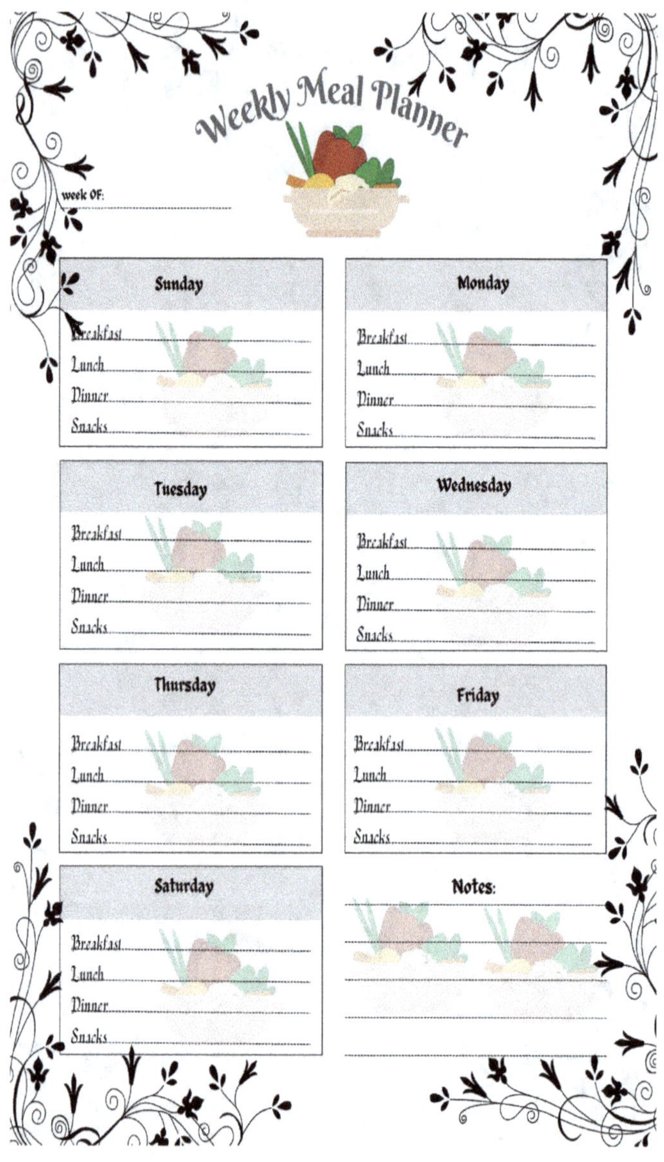

Weekly Meal Planner

week OF:

Sunday
Breakfast
Lunch
Dinner
Snacks

Monday
Breakfast
Lunch
Dinner
Snacks

Tuesday
Breakfast
Lunch
Dinner
Snacks

Wednesday
Breakfast
Lunch
Dinner
Snacks

Thursday
Breakfast
Lunch
Dinner
Snacks

Friday
Breakfast
Lunch
Dinner
Snacks

Saturday
Breakfast
Lunch
Dinner
Snacks

Notes:

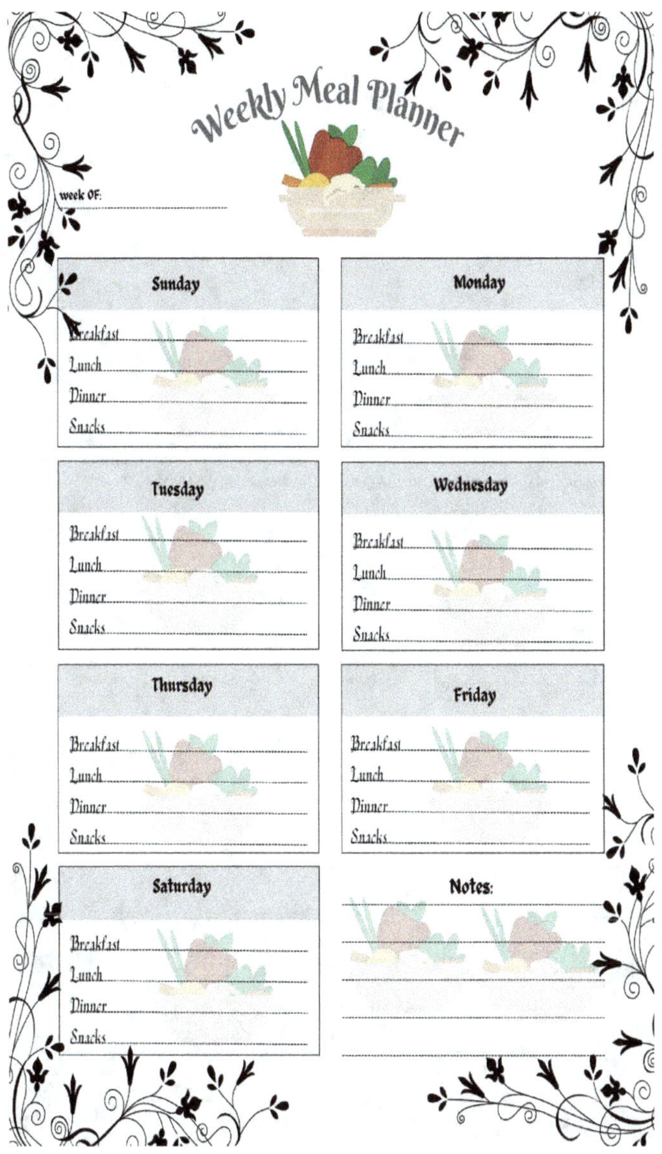

Weekly Meal Planner
week OF:

Sunday
Breakfast
Lunch
Dinner
Snacks

Monday
Breakfast
Lunch
Dinner
Snacks

Tuesday
Breakfast
Lunch
Dinner
Snacks

Wednesday
Breakfast
Lunch
Dinner
Snacks

Thursday
Breakfast
Lunch
Dinner
Snacks

Friday
Breakfast
Lunch
Dinner
Snacks

Saturday
Breakfast
Lunch
Dinner
Snacks

Notes:

Weekly Meal Planner

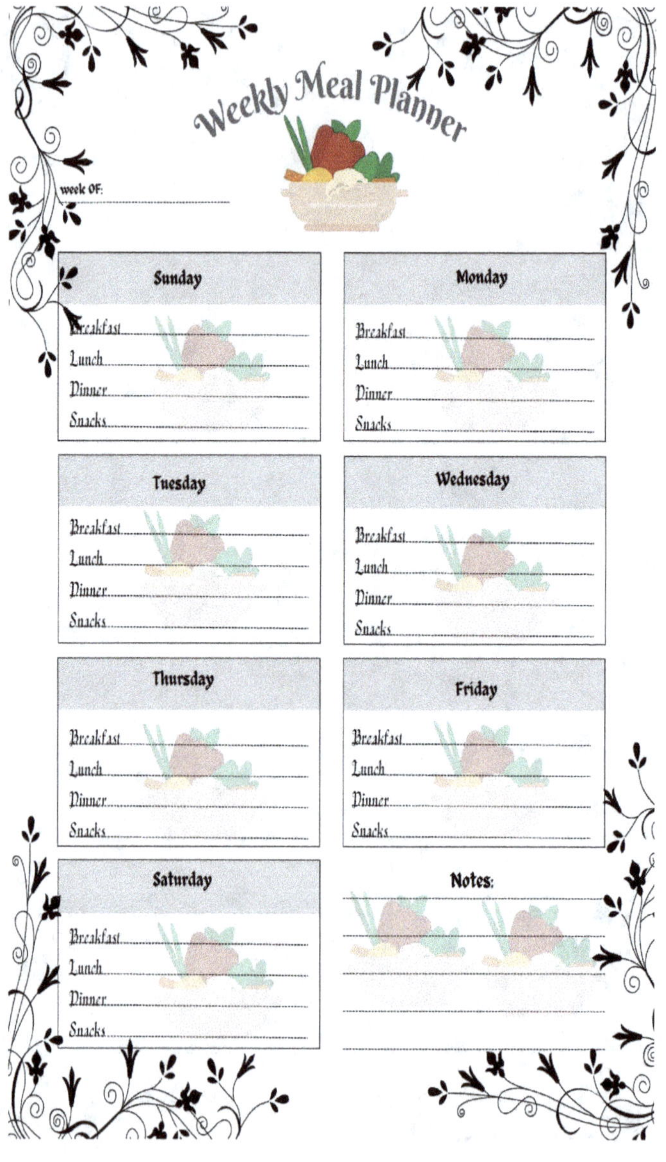

week OF: ___________________

Sunday
Breakfast ....
Lunch ....
Dinner ....
Snacks ....

Monday
Breakfast ....
Lunch ....
Dinner ....
Snacks ....

Tuesday
Breakfast ....
Lunch ....
Dinner ....
Snacks ....

Wednesday
Breakfast ....
Lunch ....
Dinner ....
Snacks ....

Thursday
Breakfast ....
Lunch ....
Dinner ....
Snacks ....

Friday
Breakfast ....
Lunch ....
Dinner ....
Snacks ....

Saturday
Breakfast ....
Lunch ....
Dinner ....
Snacks ....

Notes:

Weekly Meal Planner

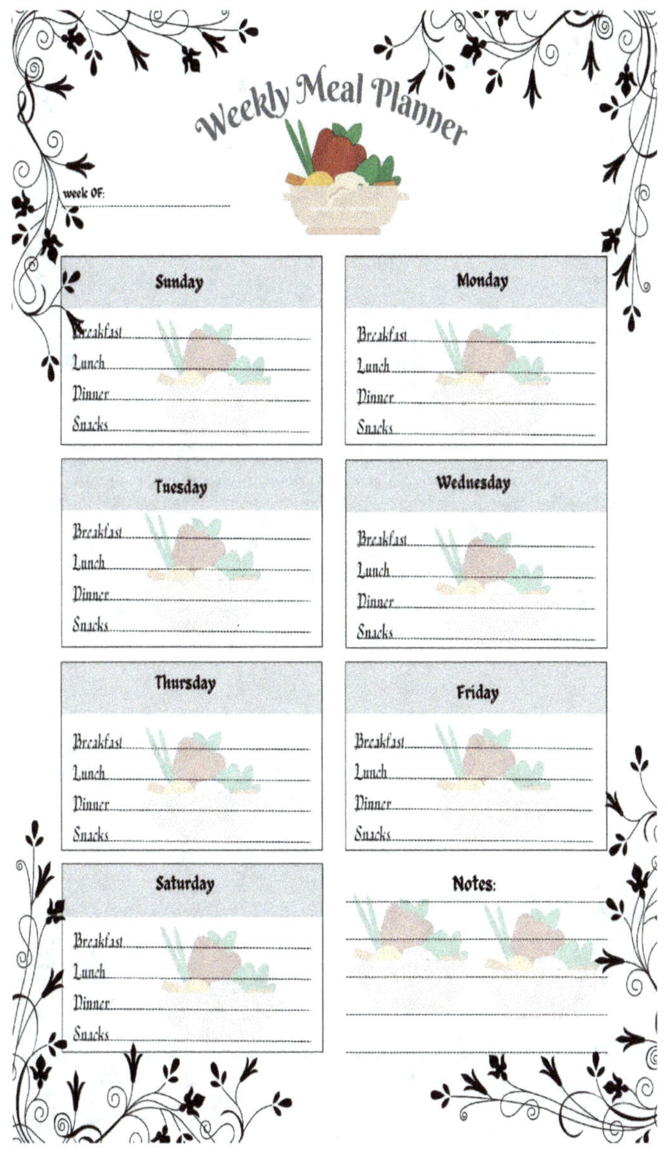

week OF: __________

Sunday
Breakfast
Lunch
Dinner
Snacks

Monday
Breakfast
Lunch
Dinner
Snacks

Tuesday
Breakfast
Lunch
Dinner
Snacks

Wednesday
Breakfast
Lunch
Dinner
Snacks

Thursday
Breakfast
Lunch
Dinner
Snacks

Friday
Breakfast
Lunch
Dinner
Snacks

Saturday
Breakfast
Lunch
Dinner
Snacks

Notes:

Weekly Meal Planner

week OF: _______________

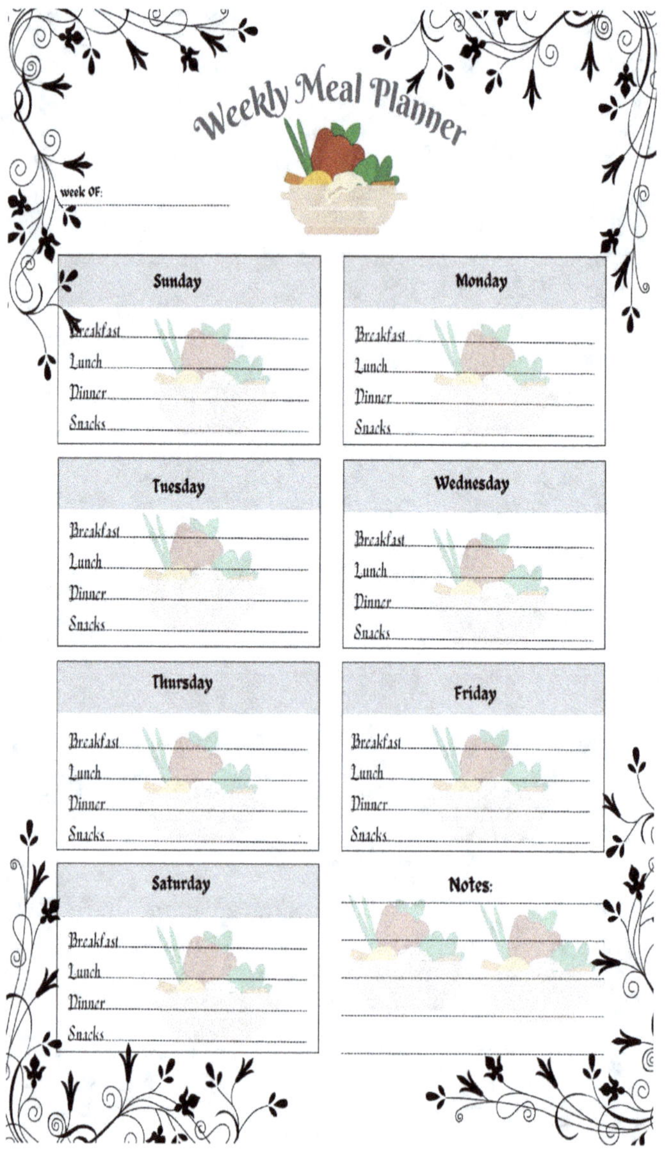

Sunday

Breakfast ....
Lunch ....
Dinner ....
Snacks ....

Monday

Breakfast ....
Lunch ....
Dinner ....
Snacks ....

Tuesday

Breakfast ....
Lunch ....
Dinner ....
Snacks ....

Wednesday

Breakfast ....
Lunch ....
Dinner ....
Snacks ....

Thursday

Breakfast ....
Lunch ....
Dinner ....
Snacks ....

Friday

Breakfast ....
Lunch ....
Dinner ....
Snacks ....

Saturday

Breakfast ....
Lunch ....
Dinner ....
Snacks ....

Notes:

Weekly Meal Planner

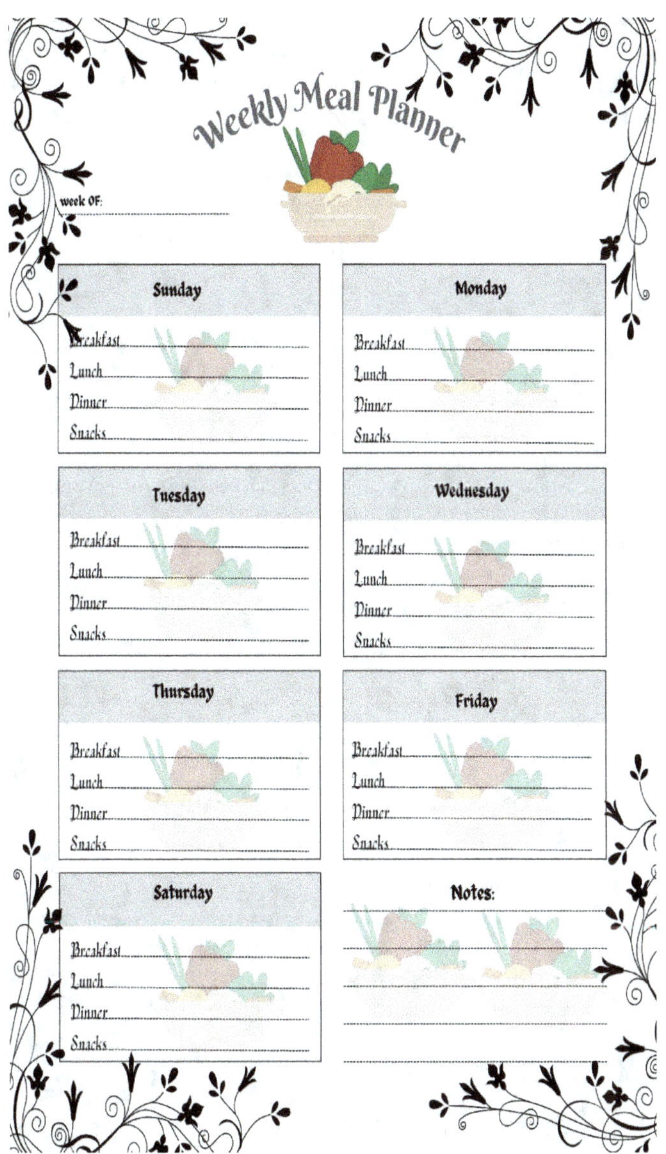

week OF: _______________

	Sunday
Breakfast	
Lunch	
Dinner	
Snacks	

	Monday
Breakfast	
Lunch	
Dinner	
Snacks	

	Tuesday
Breakfast	
Lunch	
Dinner	
Snacks	

	Wednesday
Breakfast	
Lunch	
Dinner	
Snacks	

	Thursday
Breakfast	
Lunch	
Dinner	
Snacks	

	Friday
Breakfast	
Lunch	
Dinner	
Snacks	

	Saturday
Breakfast	
Lunch	
Dinner	
Snacks	

Notes:

Weekly Meal Planner

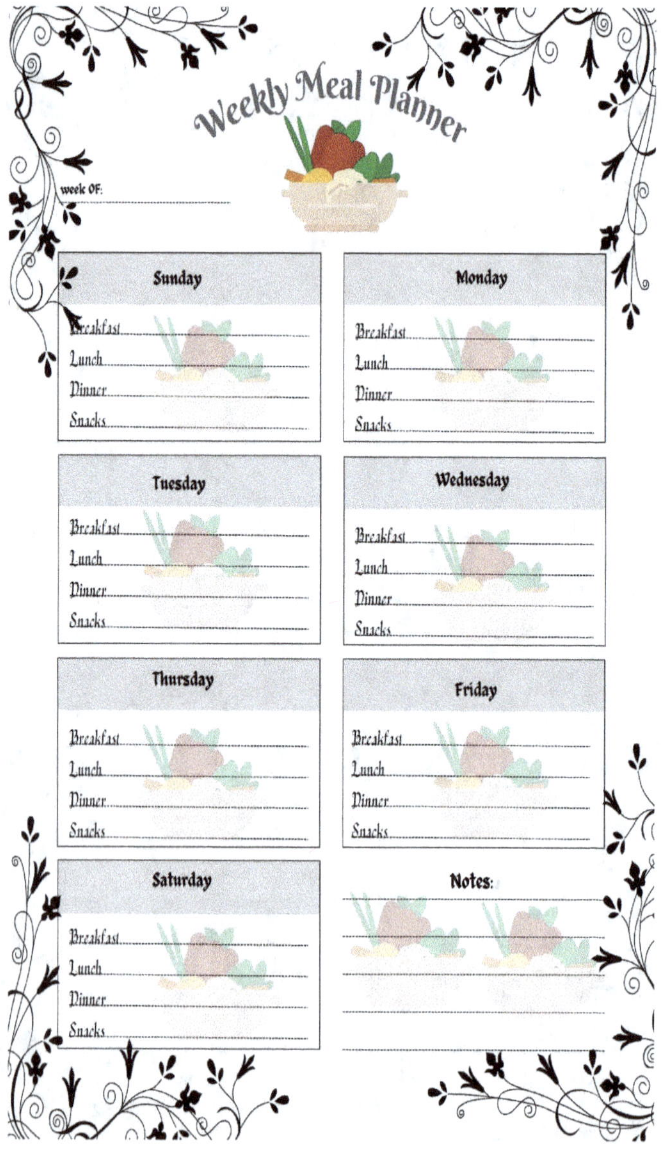

week OF: ______________________

Sunday

Breakfast ....
Lunch ....
Dinner ....
Snacks ....

Monday

Breakfast ....
Lunch ....
Dinner ....
Snacks ....

Tuesday

Breakfast ....
Lunch ....
Dinner ....
Snacks ....

Wednesday

Breakfast ....
Lunch ....
Dinner ....
Snacks ....

Thursday

Breakfast ....
Lunch ....
Dinner ....
Snacks ....

Friday

Breakfast ....
Lunch ....
Dinner ....
Snacks ....

Saturday

Breakfast ....
Lunch ....
Dinner ....
Snacks ....

Notes:

Weekly Meal Planner

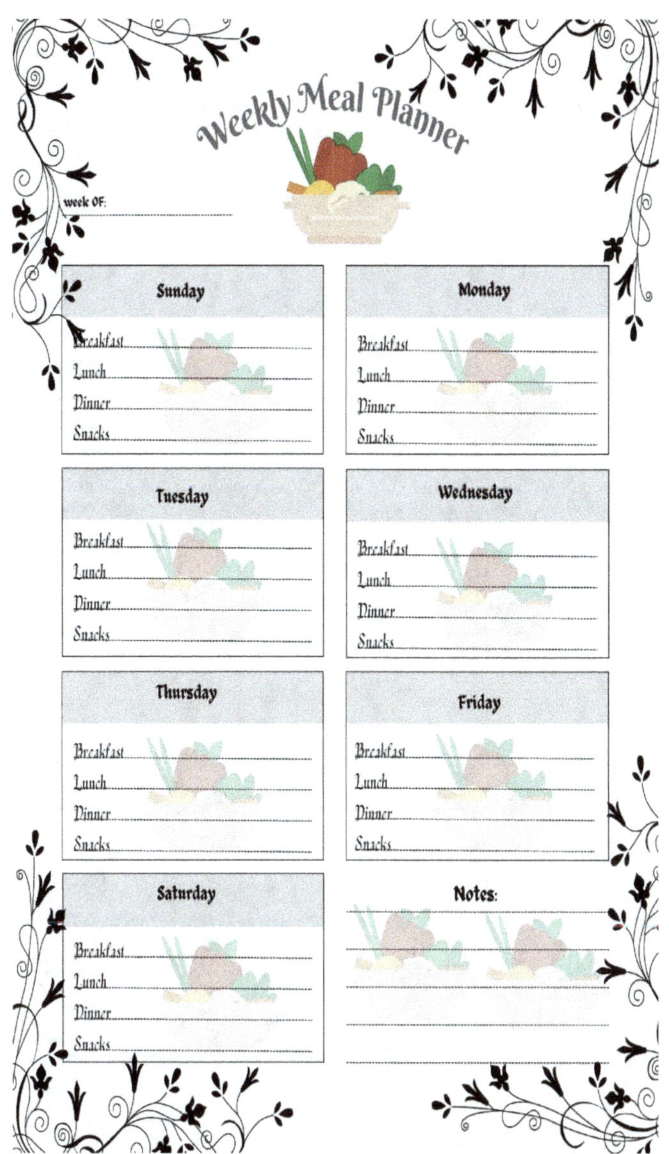

week OF: ____________________

Sunday

Breakfast ....
Lunch ....
Dinner ....
Snacks ....

Monday

Breakfast ....
Lunch ....
Dinner ....
Snacks ....

Tuesday

Breakfast ....
Lunch ....
Dinner ....
Snacks ....

Wednesday

Breakfast ....
Lunch ....
Dinner ....
Snacks ....

Thursday

Breakfast ....
Lunch ....
Dinner ....
Snacks ....

Friday

Breakfast ....
Lunch ....
Dinner ....
Snacks ....

Saturday

Breakfast ....
Lunch ....
Dinner ....
Snacks ....

Notes: